INTRINSIC

STRENGTH

TRAINING

A BREAKTHROUGH PROGRAM FOR REAL-WORLD FUNCTIONAL STRENGTH AND TRUE ATHLETIC POWER

ANGELO GRINCERI

INTRINSIC STRENGTH TRAINING

A BREAKTHROUGH PROGRAM FOR REAL-WORLD FUNCTIONAL STRENGTH AND TRUE ATHLETIC POWER

ANGELO GRINCERI

Published in the United States by: Dragon Door Publications, Inc.
5 East County Rd B, #3 • Little Canada, MN 55117
Tel: (651) 487-2180 • Fax: (651) 487-3954
Credit card orders: 1-800-899-5111 • Email: support@dragondoor.com • Website: www.dragondoor.com

ISBN-10: 1-942812-07-8   ISBN-13: 978-1-942812-07-4

This edition first published in October, 2016
Printed in China

BOOK DESIGN: Derek Brigham • www.dbrigham.com • bigd@dbrigham.com

PHOTOGRAPHY: Al Kavadlo credit for one photo on page 70

DISCLAIMER: The authors and publisher of this material are not responsible in any manner whatsoever for any injury that may occur through following the instructions contained in this material. The activities, physical and otherwise, described herein for informational purposes only, may be too strenuous or dangerous for some people and the reader(s) should consult a physician before engaging in them. The content of this book is for informational and educational purposes only and should not be considered medical advice, diagnosis, or treatment. Readers should not disregard, or delay in obtaining, medical advice for any medical condition they may have, and should seek the assistance of their health care professionals for any such conditions because of information contained within this publication.

— TABLE OF CONTENTS —

FOREWORD:

By Gary Gray V

INTRODUCTION 1

SECTION 1 - Out with the Old in with the New

Chapter 1:   We Need a New Approach to an Old Concept 7

                 How Did Exercise Regress to Sitting and Standing Still? 9

                 Why Intrinsic Strength Training is Superior 11

Chapter 2:   You Have a Choice 13

                 Are You All Show and No Go? 15

Chapter 3:   Stop Selling Yourself Short 23

                 A Fundamental Fitness Failure 23

SESTION 2 - Life is NOT Stationary

Chapter 4:   Pieces Move Together to Move the Whole 33

Chapter 5:   The Core Does More 39

Chapter 6:   Full Body Functions 47

Chapter 7:   Protecting the Body from the Inside Out 61

Chapter 8:   Walking with Force 67

SECTION 3 - Taking Control of the Problem

Chapter 9:   We Are Only as Strong as Our Weakest Link 81

Chapter 10:   With Repetition Comes Replication 87

Chapter 11:   Involving More of the Core with Upright Exercise 93

Chapter 12:   The 10 Commandments of Intrinsic Strength Training 97

Section 4 - Intrinsic Strength Training Exercises

CHEST—Creating a Compatible Chest 131

BACK—Beneficial Workout 149

SHOULDER—Symmetrical Shoulders 177

LEGS—Limitless Legs 211

ARMS—Articulating Arms 235

CORE—Abdominal Focus 263

Section 5 - Sample Exercise Combinations, Circuits, and Weekly Workout Splits

SAMPLE EXERCISE COMBINATIONS 275

SAMPLE CIRCUITS 276

SAMPLE WEEKLY WORKOUT SPLITS 278

About The Author 284

FOREWORD

BY DR. GARY GRAY, PT, FAFS

Understanding the "why" behind the "what" provides competence and confidence in our lives. Instead of just being told what to do, we appreciate and benefit greatly from being told why we should do something a certain way. The wisdom and beauty of ***Intrinsic Strength Training*** lies in the logical way Angelo Grinceri provides the why behind the what.

Angelo does a masterful job of presenting the truths and principles of how our human body functions, and from those principles develops powerful strategies that provide the foundation for the abundant techniques (movements/exercises) presented. As a result, we develop ongoing competence and confidence in what we are doing and in our own abilities because we are empowered with the "why" behind the "what".

Angelo presents his own personal journey from a period of training with artificial, isolated, non-functional exercises to authentic, integrated, and functional exercises that have transformed his body and therefore his life. Moving and feeling "like a lethargic uncoordinated moose", Angelo realized he needed a dramatic change. As a result he dedicated himself to learning and understanding everything he possibly could about our miraculous and wonderful human body.

Within that journey—which is ongoing for Angelo and for all of us—I had the privilege of getting to know Angelo as he studied Applied Functional Science® with us at Gray Institute®, ultimately becoming a Fellow of Applied Functional Science®. Not only did I grow to appreciate Angelo's incredible mind full of knowledge, but appreciated even more so his heart and spirit full of passion. The success of ***Intrinsic Strength Training*** is due to Angelo's experience with his own body, his openness with his own mind and his spiritual caring.

You will greatly appreciate Angelo's 10 Commandments of Intrinsic Strength Training®. They provide us a comprehensive summary of the principles and strategies utilized to justify his full-body, integrated, multi-directional approach to resistance training. Angelo presents a refreshing description of the body's core, thus revealing that the core is everything from the nose to the toes and is influenced and developed through movements of the hands and feet simultaneously.

All the exercises presented in **Intrinsic Strength Training** allow for improving our ability to move and control our body, and are logically categorized to facilitate building and training desired muscle groups. Each grouping of exercises includes real life examples of the integrated movements, further enhancing our understanding of the "why" behind the "what". Each exercise is beautifully presented and illustrated with pictures, easy-to-follow descriptions, and a bonus section entitled Angelo's Advice. There is nothing better than to benefit from the personal experience of someone who is successful in what he does.

You will thoroughly enjoy Angelo's wonderful work of purpose and passion. You, too, will appreciate Angelo's wisdom, recognize the transformation of his body, and become thankful for his sharing from the heart. Because of Angelo's devotion and dedication, we all can experience this opportunity to "restore life to our entire body." It is an honor for me to introduce **Intrinsic Strength Training** to you, as well as to consider Angelo a friend and mentor.

—Gary Gray

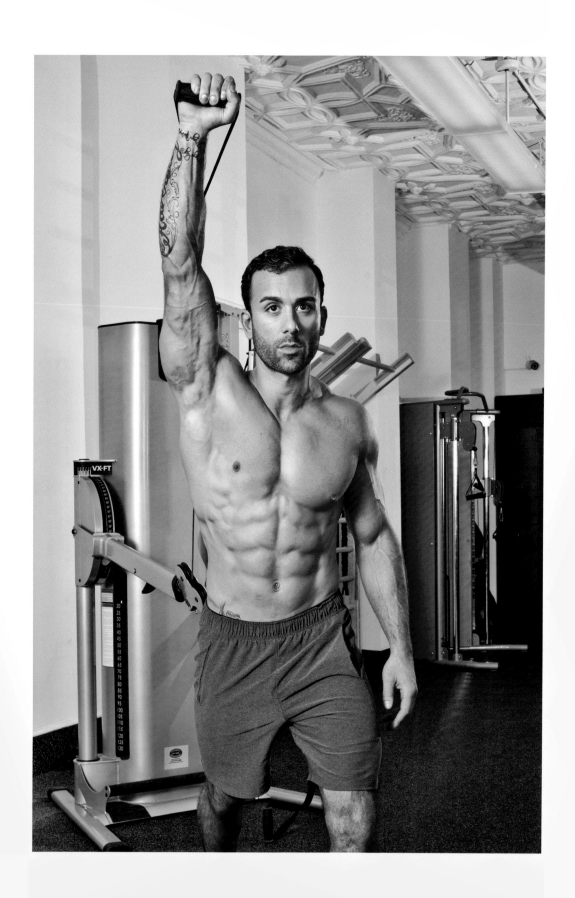

INTRODUCTION

Intrinsic Strength Training® is the product of 5,000+ hours of personal exercise experience, 2,000+ hours of education, and 8,000+ hours of professional personal and group training. Over the last 12 years I have dedicated my life to experimenting and researching every well-known exercise type. I've taken on various fitness focused lifestyles, each providing me with different aesthetic and physically-able versions of myself. With these differing fitness regimens, I've experienced different pros and cons from embracing each lifestyle. Over time, following a bodybuilding regimen provided me with aesthetic pros as well as athletic cons. A conventional body building training regimen left me feeling stiff and lethargic when required to move throughout the day. While conventional cross training would provide me with a more athletic body, I was unable to reach the aesthetic goals that I desired.

On the other hand, I've also lived through getting hurt and being inactive. Challenging me to start back from square 1 on multiple occasions. This personal journey through the depths of fitness and wellness have lead me to formulate innovative and effective exercises, life-changing stretch routines, and an easily achievable healthy lifestyle.

Intrinsic Strength Training® will challenge and improve your ability to move and control your body while building and toning your desired muscle group. In my 10,000+ hours in wellness and fitness, I have found that this evolutionary approach to stationary resistance training is what works best.

Seated resistance training is a flawed concept and will not create or reinforce the full body integration needed to experience some of the best joys in life. When exercise is limited to repetitive movements performed while seated, lying down, or standing still, the body will only get better at sitting, lying down, or standing still. Conventional seated and stationary exercise restricts dynamic, full body movements and provides artificial stability to most of the body while only training a few specific muscles at a time.

Do you really want to spend precious gym time reinforcing the bad physical habits of the work day, or would you rather use that time to prepare the body for a full life of movement?

Children and adults remain fit, healthy and pain-free by living a life full of movement. They live active lifestyles that challenge their entire bodies all day, every day. Throughout the day, we move our entire body as one integrated unit even while simply walking from place to place. Every fun physical activity as well as most chores around the house and yard, require full body movements.

Many people today have the gift—and curse—of a sedentary work environment. In a typical office setting, physical activity is limited and the vast majority of the workday is spent sitting. Since our bodies are designed to adapt to whatever we repetitively do, our muscles, tendons, and nervous systems will adapt to this habitually seated position. This brings us to an important question—why are many classic resistance training exercises performed while sitting or lying down on a bench or machine? The more time we spend with any activity, the more we will improve at that specific activity. So, why would we want to only be our best while sitting?

If you've recently searched the Internet for health and wellness information, you may have noticed that there is a "war on sitting" and a prevalence of phrases like "sitting is the new smoking". You probably already know that constantly sitting is not good for you, may lead to poor posture, or that it will make some of your muscles too tight. While no one should believe everything on the Internet, these particular sentiments are grounded in truth. A lifestyle dominated by prolonged sitting can contribute to many unwanted health issues. These issues can include a slouched posture, muscle imbalances, a weak core, low back pain, a lack of physical coordination, and a higher risk for serious cardiovascular problems. With this information, it's no surprise that many health-conscious individuals hit the gym to combat these negative effects. Plus, working out on a regular basis will burn more calories, build more muscle and improve heart function.

Ideally, a workout should not only improve your physique, but should also help improve your balance, coordination, and precise body control. This led to the innovative approach to exercise called Intrinsic Strength Training®. Instead of boring stationary exercises, the Intrinsic Strength Training® program requires the entire body to work together during each and every exercise, restoring life to your entire body.

Why don't we exercise in the same way that we actually move?

For example:
• Pushing or pulling open a door.
• Playing with or chasing after your children.
• Exploring an unpaved path to enjoy an excellent view or sunset.
• Helping someone out of a dangerous situation.

All of these tasks or situations require simultaneous arm and leg movements, and they dynamically challenge the body as one integrated unit.

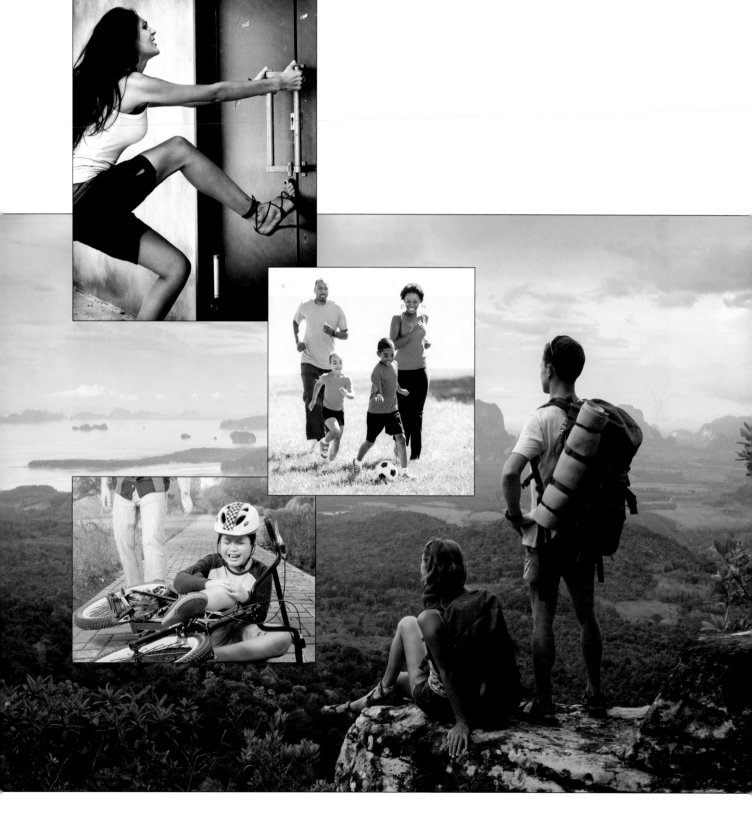

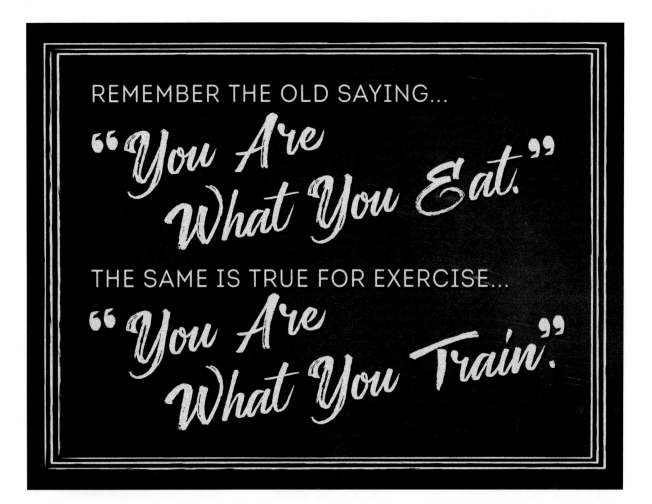

REMEMBER THE OLD SAYING...

"You Are What You Eat."

THE SAME IS TRUE FOR EXERCISE...

"You Are What You Train".

Intrinsic Strength Training® invites you to start moving and earn the muscle tone and body control you have always wanted by stepping away from the stationary, lethargic, artificial, and disconnected approach to resistance training.

OUT
WITH THE OLD
IN
WITH THE NEW

CHAPTER 1

We Need a New Approach to an Old Concept

Intrinsic Strength Training® is a modern upgrade of classic resistance training. This new approach to muscle isolation requires the entire body to work as a single, integrated unit. This upgraded system assures symmetrical and balanced physique improvements. Each IST exercise incorporates the entire body and activates more muscles, toning your physique faster and more efficiently than classic resistance training. IST burns more calories, improves full body strength, coordination, stability, balance and movement literacy. *After using IST, you will look and feel like a superior version of yourself.*

On the other hand, I've also lived through getting hurt and being inactive. Challenging me to start back from square 1 on multiple occasions. This personal journey through the depths of fitness and wellness have lead me to formulate innovative and effective exercises, life-changing stretch routines, and an easily achievable healthy lifestyle.

Intrinsic Strength Training® will challenge and improve your ability to move and control your body while building and toning your desired muscle group. In my 10,000+ hours in wellness and fitness, I have found that this evolutionary approach to stationary resistance training is what works best.

This upgraded approach to exercise will challenge anyone from the seasoned athlete and weekend warrior to the everyday beginner looking to build a strong foundation.

How could seated exercise possibly be the best approach? The comfy seat, machine, or padded bench allows multiple parts of the body to rest while requiring other parts to work much differently than when standing upright. This type of assistance and isolation can cause enormous problems. In the real world outside the gym, we never have the assistance of a chair to help us with the physical activities and demands of life. We will never find physical success when we let the other half of the body rest.

What's really the difference?

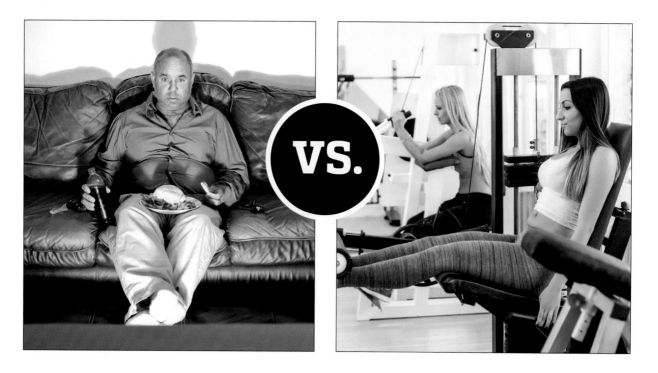

Think of all the exercises you've spent countless hours performing. How much of that time was spent working out while sitting down or standing still?

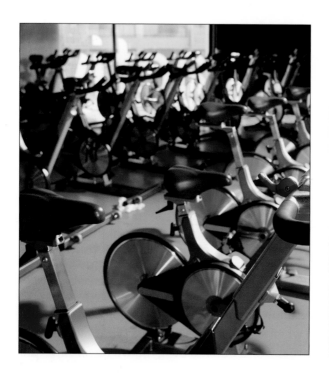

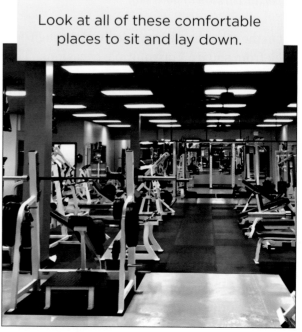

Look at all of these comfortable places to sit and lay down.

INTRINSIC STRENGTH TRAINING

How Did Exercise Regress to Sitting and Standing Still?

The problem began when mainstream fitness embraced bodybuilding culture and began to sell stationary individual muscle isolation exercises to the average American. Over the past thirty years, many fitness gurus and personal trainers perpetuated the belief that faster weight loss was best achieved by building more muscle to increase the body's caloric requirements. A body with more muscle will require more energy to operate than a body with less muscle mass. Compare a V8 to a four-cylinder engine, the bigger engine will consume and require more gasoline (energy).

You may have heard "all you have to do is turn your fat into muscle." While this sounds reasonable, it's impossible to turn a fat cell into a muscle cell. That quote originated from a study which found that one pound of muscle can burn up to six and a half calories per day. This created the idea that more muscle would burn more calories, and drove the focus of general fitness towards isolated muscle-building exercises. The bodybuilding world preached that stationary isolated exercise was the fastest path to creating the best looking physiques. They claimed that exercisers could shed pounds of unwanted fat simply by building up each muscle individually. New gym goers quickly put on a few pounds of muscle following the concept of isolated resistance training. It was easy to see how the rapid aesthetic changes from this segmented approach to exercise became very popular very quickly.

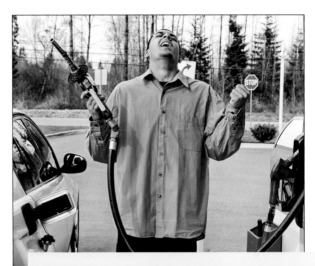

Just like an 8 cylinder vehicle will use more gas than a 4 cylinder, using more gas—more muscle—requires more energy, and the body will use more calories throughout the day.

However, I will show you that lethargic isolated exercise and machine-based training is not the only answer—and more importantly, that it is not the best choice.

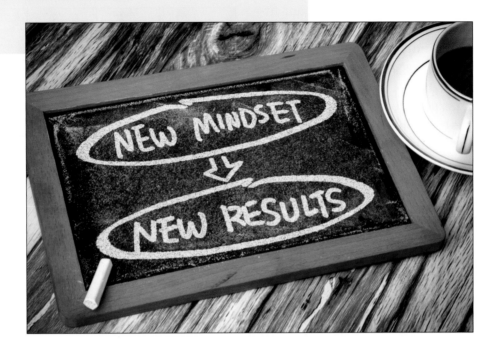

Intrinsic Strength Training®️ will revolutionize your approach to resistance training and quickly transform your body. When compared to conventional resistance training exercises, IST will provide you with many more benefits including a superior way to improve general health, build lean muscle, improve full body control, balance, coordination, as well as create useful strength, and burn unwanted body fat.

The key to a stronger, smarter and more symmetrical body is to use the entire body with each part of every exercise. Simply put, Intrinsic Strength Training®️ recognizes that bodies are designed to work as one complete integrated unit. "The Entire Body Every Time" (TEBET) is an easy way to remember this concept. Each IST exercise was created with TEBET in mind by continually challenging all of the body's many parts to work together. Every upright movement requires the lower extremities (legs), the upper extremities (arms and head), and the core (everything

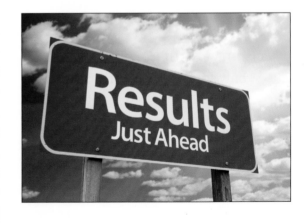

in-between—hips, spine, and shoulders) to work together as one interdependent unit. The simple act of walking requires the involvement of every muscle in the body. If you place your hands on your legs, butt, and torso, you can feel how all of these muscles engage differently with each step.

With each Intrinsic Strength Training® exercise, fitness enthusiasts of all levels can challenge their entire bodies to change positions while focusing on contracting (eccentrically and concentrically) designated muscle groups. *Imagine using your favorite resistance training exercise to target a desired muscle group while dynamically challenging the entire body to maintain steady and safe upright positions while continually stepping.*

By continually challenging the body to work as one integrated unit during these upright movements, you will improve your balance, coordination, and ability to control your body. This will directly and immediately improve core stability and strength, muscular symmetry, joint health, strength, and posture. IST provides the aesthetic benefits of following a bodybuilding training regimen with the athleticism and health benefits of three-dimensional movement training as needed in day to day life.

IST workouts will bring you one step closer to unlocking your full athletic and aesthetic potential. Build a body as strong and powerful as a gorilla which can also move as fluidly as a ballerina.

Intrinsic Strength Training® is superior—both physiologically and biomechanically—to traditional stationary and seated resistance (weight) training.

Intrinsic Strength Training® will rebuild your foundation.
- Excessively sedentary lifestyles weaken our foundations and make our bodies more prone to injury and pain. Dynamic upright resistance training is perfect for a beginner or someone returning to exercise after an injury. This training challenges and improves the body's foundation and upright function.

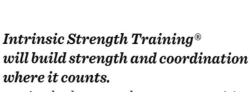

Intrinsic Strength Training® will build strength and coordination where it counts.

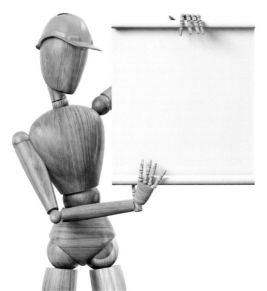

- As the lower and upper extremities are challenged while moving simultaneously with each exercise, full-body coordination will improve. IST's three-dimensional exercises replicate many of our physical requirements throughout the day. In a typical day, we are required to move, so improving our ability to move well will enhance daily life and decrease the chance of injury.

Intrinsic Strength Training® will guide you to a symmetrical physique.

- By requiring the whole body to work together with each exercise, each muscle will get an equal amount of work, resulting in an evenly trained and developed physique. This dynamic, upright, and unilateral approach to resistance training produces a stronger physique, with even muscle tone—leaving weak and underdeveloped muscle groups nowhere to hide.

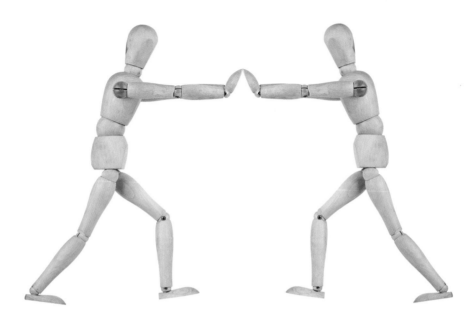

Intrinsic Strength Training® is a smarter use of your time.

- Regularly changing the body's position while moving the arms and legs simultaneously will require every muscle in the body to stay stimulated. If more muscles remain active during every exercise, the body will use more energy—and burn more calories—as compared to seated and machine-based resistance training exercises. More importantly, these dynamic exercises will challenge your ability to control your body. Improving this ability directly improves your balance, coordination, and dynamic stability—which is required for all locomotion.

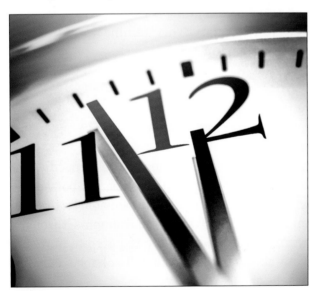

While walking down the street, if you can avoid someone running towards you (without stopping or losing your balance while continuing on your original path) then you've successfully used dynamic stability.

CHAPTER 2

You Have the Choice

Growing up, I would daydream about having the physique of a modern day superhero. I grew up idolizing Arnold Schwarzenegger, Lou Ferrigno (Incredible Hulk), Sylvester Stallone (Rocky & Rambo), and of course 8x Mr. Olympia Ronnie Coleman.

After years of replicating their bodybuilding training regimens, I certainly looked like a superhero.

But looks can be deceiving.

I remember looking strong, but I only felt strong while doing stationary "strength training and muscle building" exercises on a chair or on a machine. I had no sense of balance or precise body control, and certainly no core strength. My posture was horrible, my muscles and joints were tight, and even though I looked strong as hell, I moved like a lethargic, uncoordinated moose!

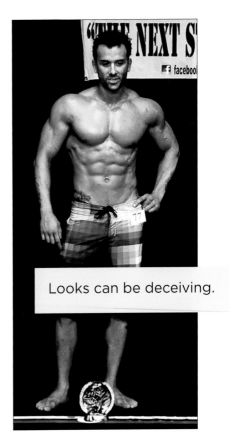

Looks can be deceiving.

Eventually, I realized none of the strength I had inside the gym translated into real useable strength anywhere else. Outside the gym, simple chores and physical activities, requiring various types of reaching and stepping, would conquer me. Inside the gym, I would conquer every basic lift and machine. Filling a bar up with plates and repping out an entire stack of weights on a machine was easy. I could easily load up the leg press machine with as many plates as possible. I could easily bench over 375lb for reps, and rep out bent over rows with more than 275lb. For about six years, I trained by sitting on my ass, standing still, and mindlessly forcing out extremely limited, assisted reps. Many times I'd only train in one position through a very specific, limited range of motion.

While I was competing in the NPC (National Physique Committee), my goals were to build muscle and burn fat. I spent countless hours researching every method of getting better, faster results, but kept finding the same information. Every bodybuilder, fitness model, and celebrity trainer who had an amazing physique would say to use isolated resistance exercises with rep ranges for strength or hypertrophy. They were always pictured doing an exercise on a machine, bench, or chair that provided some support or assistance. None of these athletes mentioned the adverse effects of continuously training the body in such an unnatural, segmented way. Some of the bodybuilders would mention including at least one "complex lift" with each workout for full body muscle-building (squat, deadlift, and bench press). Sometimes a pull-up, push-up, or overhead shoulder press were mentioned, and while these are great exercises with multiple benefits, they still have limited movement complexity.

None of these aesthetic gurus ever mentioned the importance of training the body as a dynamic, integrated unit.

What was MY training missing?

Improve your life and challenge yourself by creating a body from the inside out with Intrinsic Strength Training®. IST focuses on enhancing full body strength, balance, movement literacy, muscle tone, and creating an amazing core—results with rewards inside and outside the gym.

I achieved excellent aesthetic results, but none of it translated into truly functional, useable strength during my chores and play. I was "all show and no go". I worked out all the time but simple physical tasks outside the gym were still very difficult. I was not as strong as I looked, and that pissed me off! I began to feel cheated when I realized the bodybuilding protocols were actually hindering my "real world" physical abilities and experiences outside the gym. I knew something was missing in my approach to exercise, and with this realization I began to create Intrinsic Strength Training®.

I realized that my big muscles and ripped six pack abs were aesthetically pleasing, but not very functional. I was shocked to realize that maxing out most of the weight machines and using heavy weights for squatting, deadlifting, and benching failed to provide me with the usable strength and efficiency for many activities I chose to do outside the gym. This limited approach to fitness with seated and stationary exercises failed to integrate my interconnected body parts and left my core extremely weak. With this training, I was only comfortable, confident and secure while sitting down or standing still (and as stiff as possible).

Even though I never once stopped working on my abs, I experienced having a "weak core" on many occasions. It surprised me every time. For years, I had trained each section of my body using the most highly regarded, traditional methods—and I NEVER skipped an abdominal workout of sit ups and crunches! But with such a weak core and little experience moving into different upright positions, my athleticism and coordination certainly did not match my looks.

"A chain is only as strong as its weakest link".

An entire structure can be affected by one weak part. Similarly, the entire body is only as strong as its weakest segment.

Is your body's potential limited by a weak core?

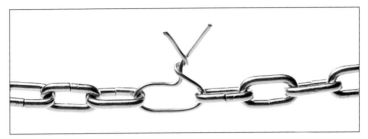

My ability to generate integrated strength, have full control over my body, and balance in various upright positions was below subpar—especially for a dedicated gym goer who considered himself to be "Mr. Fitness".

How is your core strength?

You might also suffer from a weak core, or have poor abilities to integrate the strength of your entire body. The following are a few examples of activities that made me realize that my time spent in the gym was not beneficial to my active dynamic lifestyle.

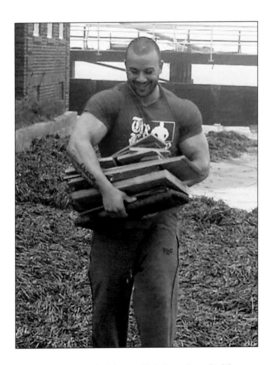

Helping my father with yard work: As a narcissistic teenager who consistently lifted weights every day for a few years. With added muscle weight, I thought I was pretty strong and badass. I was excited to try and out-do my father while helping him mulch the plant beds around the house. But after only ten minutes, I was struggling to get the job done. I could barely hold on to a few bags of heavy mulch. My father looked over and said, "All that work in the gym, and you can't even carry a few bags of mulch!" While trying to carry the bags from the truck, I was quickly out of breath and my body was compensating for the load, instead of efficiently distributing the weight through my core. As the load became unbearable, I began to excessively arch my back which put unnecessary strain on my lower back. With a lack of coordination and integration, I waddled like a duck while my old man carried the bags with ease.

Please note that my dad did not spend hours lifting weights every week like I did, but he did have great full body strength from years of working on a farm and remaining active. He grew up doing real-world physical work using his entire body every time.

In spite of my awesome six pack, my core was too weak and my body control was too inefficient to distribute the weight properly for a physical task that required me to lift and move. Then, to add injury to insult, I was so sore the next day—and my father was completely fine. I wondered how could this be! I remember feeling like an ass!

Playing in Central Park: A few years ago, one of my friends challenged me to a foot race through the trails of Central Park. This impromptu race course had a few steps we needed to jump over while running. Each set of stairs only had three little steps, which didn't seem that bad. As we were racing, we both jumped across the steps. When I landed, I felt an unpleasant jolt right into my lower back as my feet slammed onto the ground. Clearly, my core musculature was not efficiently distributing the impact from my lower body. My seated and stationary approach to strength training had not prepared my legs and core to work as one.

Opening a Heavy Door: Have you ever had difficulty pushing or pulling a door open? I have. Pushing a door requires us to push with our arms while we are stepping forward with our legs. This combined task requires satisfactory full body and core integration. When I was all jacked up—while oblivious of my weak core—I struggled with this simple task time after time. While my feet kept walking forward, my arms pressed into the door which only caused my upper body to bend backward. Instead, my core should have linked my upper and lower body together to form a braced, integrated structure. A core built from heavy bench pressing could not keep me from looking like a total weakling when the door wouldn't budge.

Overhead Shoulder Pressing—With Correct Form: Anyone trying to build big, round, broad shoulders usually does some type of overhead pressing exercise. Most people do shoulder presses while seated, and sadly I was one of them. The first time I tried this exercise while standing, it was much harder. I walked to the rack and grabbed the same weighted bar I used for the seated version, then unsuccessfully tried to press the bar up and over my head. While my arms were able to lift the weight, my core could not control my body's position. I found it hard to control my muscular tension from my upper body through the core and into the floor. I began to feel the full force of the weight compress into the lower region of my back, my lumbar spine. I tried with all my might to engage my core, align my joints, and distribute the weight evenly through my entire body. However, I failed miserably. Without core control, my body was never able to find an efficient, safe joint alignment. I was forced to use a significantly lighter weight to perform the exercise safely with control and proper joint alignment—and without discomfort in my lower back. Even with a lighter weight, it was still challenging.

Something was missing from my training. If I was able to lift a weight while seated, why couldn't I do it while standing upright? My body had no idea how to integrate the effort successfully because I had spent years training my body to work only in individual segments. This was the last straw! My training needed to change for my own safety and quality of life. By changing the fundamental philosophy and execution of my workout routine, Intrinsic Strength Training® was born.

If you spend most of your day sitting, performing seated exercises, using the machines, and avoiding the challenge of training your body through upright positions, you most likely also have a weak and unstable and core.

A more confident body = more memorable life experiences

Just a few years later, a personal adventure of mine required full body integration, confidence and serious strength. While backpacking through the island of Ibiza, Spain, I came across a secluded local beach with crystal clear water surrounded by a beautiful rock landscape. Fifty meters into the water was a rock formation with a cliff. A group of local adults and children were laughing as they swam to the cliff, climbed on top and jumped off, over and over again. I decided to swim out to it, but there was a catch. Only after I swam to the formation did I notice that I would have to climb up and over forty feet of boulders to reach the top of the cliff. There was no easy path to the top.

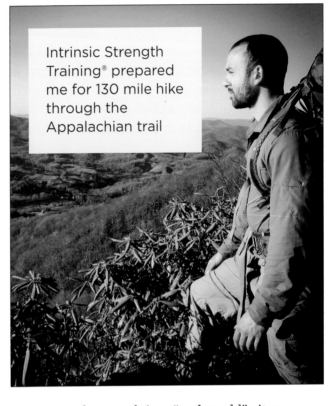

Intrinsic Strength Training® prepared me for 130 mile hike through the Appalachian trail

Because of Intrinsic Strength Training®'s full-body multi-directional approach to resistance training, I felt extremely confident in my abilities to swim, climb, and jump—even though I didn't spend much time swimming as a child. Even after a 50-meter swim, the climb seemed relatively easy. I was extremely proud of myself, I was using my newly improved strength in a "real world" situation and it felt marvelous. The view from the top of the cliff—a beautiful landscape, crystal clear water, yachts, girls in bikinis—was unforgettable. After the amazing experience of jumping in, I remember watching a man with huge muscles (he was clearly a bodybuilder) attempt the same challenge. I automatically assumed he would have a hard time because he probably trains while sitting, like most bodybuilders. I watched him struggle and nearly drown during the swim. In retrospect, I should have offered to help him. After this very muscular man exerted all of his energy to swim in an extremely inefficient way, of course he failed to climb to the top of the cliff. He was having a hard time coordinating and moving his upper and lower limbs to climb up the rock face. After realizing he wouldn't be

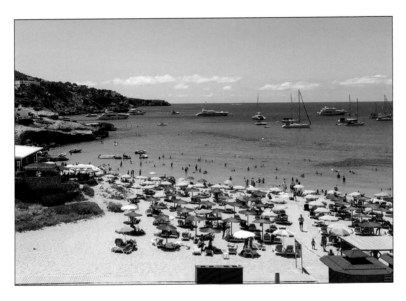

able to climb up the cliff, he headed back down to the beach. He was forced to accept that his lack of physical ability kept him from having an amazing, memorable experience.

He trained himself to sit and that is how he ended up spending his entire vacation!

All of these experiences are examples of how years of bodybuilding training robbed me and many others of true strength, body control, and athletic potential. I wasn't able to help my father, I lost a race, I had back pain, and a door kicked my ass. However, after rebuilding my body with a new approach to training, I was able to have an unforgettable experience on vacation. Not only did cliff jumping turn into a great workout, it left me with a natural body high that lasted all day. I felt confident in my own body's strength, and fully alive as my inner child came out to play!

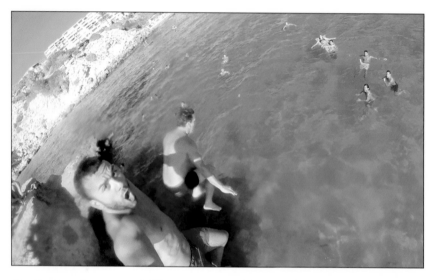

How well you can control your body can be crucial for getting out of a dangerous situation, avoiding a fall or avoiding other potential injuries throughout your day to day life.

Your body is designed to operate as a fully interconnected unit that MOVES freely. Exercise which respects the body as an interconnected, integrated unit that moves is an absolute necessity. Improving your ability to move and control your body will drastically improve your daily life with less physical struggle, chance of injury, and less joint instability. Most importantly, this type of training inspires self confidence.

Consider some of the physically challenging tasks of a typical week:

- Picking up your child/pet, or picking up a mess that your child/pet has made will require a step and reach towards the floor.
- Putting the groceries away on shelves or in cabinets usually requires a step and reach across, above, below, or behind the body.
- Pulling or pushing a door open will always require the combination of a step and a pull or push.

These simple tasks require coordination, and for the body to move as one integrated unit.

Any physically challenging situation will almost always require the entire body to move through different positions. Another similarity between the physically challenging tasks listed above is arm movement accompanied by leg movement and vice versa.

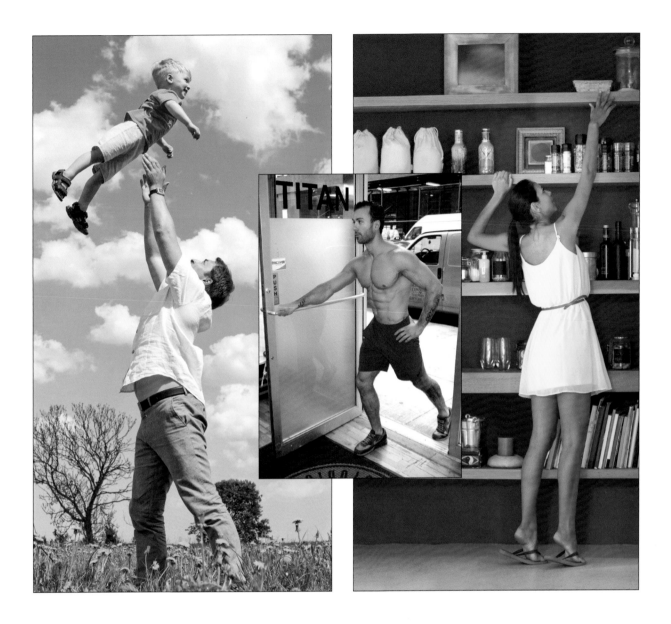

Even in a sedentary lifestyle, these everyday tasks require the upper and lower extremities to work together. Our time spent in the gym needs to prepare our bodies to handle our physical requirements. Exercise needs to not only improve our physique, but improve our abilities, safety, health and longevity over time.

Most gym goers want to improve their aesthetics, and having an aesthetic goal is great motivation. However, developing our athletic abilities is just as important. Training our bodies to look a certain way can often result in neglecting our true physical needs.

Your approach to exercise also needs to challenge and stimulate every body part.

Full body training improves full body strength, joint integration, muscular symmetry, coordination, and physical safety. The body must be trained to work as one integrated unit successfully while using resistance. When we train to handle and distribute excessive forces throughout the body as it moves, there is less chance of excessive wear and tear on the joints, directly increasing our physical longevity. Building a symmetrical physique banishes imbalances and poor posture. Most importantly, as your coordination, balance, and body control improves, your ability to trust and challenge your body improves, usually leading to new physical experiences.

Intrinsic Strength Training® provides a middle ground for enhancing the control of your own body while building and toning the muscle groups you want to improve. IST combines the aesthetics you want to see in the mirror with the athleticism your body—and lifestyle—needs.

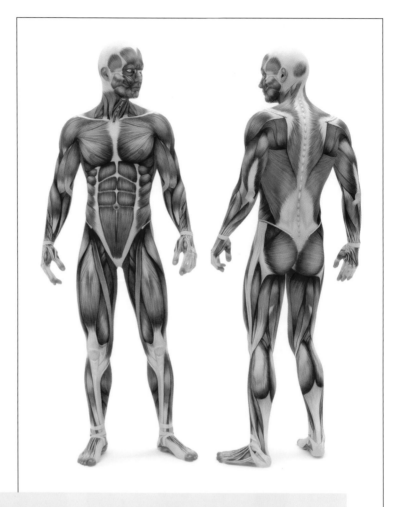

Intrinsic Strength Training® provides the best of both worlds by focusing on individual muscle groups while challenging how well you can move your whole body. The simultaneous integration of the lower and upper extremities continuously challenges the core. Each of IST's dynamic upright unilateral exercises improve athletic abilities as well as aesthetics, enhancing the ability to control your own body while symmetrically improving your physique.)

The Truth...

Human survival relies on how well we adapt to our tasks and surroundings. Simply put, we get better at what we spend time doing. Our bodies and brains are designed to remember, learn, and adapt to what we constantly and consistently do.

Which one of these three things are you interested in improving? Would you rather be really good at sitting, standing still or moving?

If you want to adapt your body for sitting, then spend more time sitting.

If you want to adapt your body to standing still, then spend more time standing still.

If you want to optimize your body for moving and meeting life's challenges, then spend more time moving!

Question your own approach to fitness. Does your current workout mimic the dynamic demands of life by stepping between different foot positions while reaching and lifting?

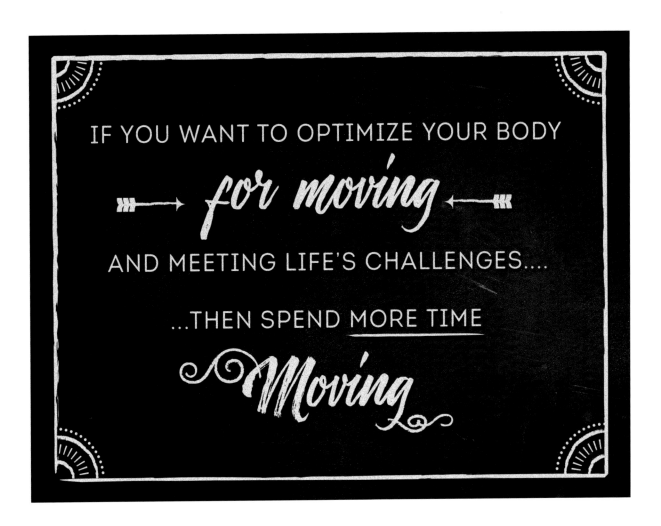

CHAPTER 3

Stop Selling Yourself Short

W e all have different fitness goals. You may be interested in losing weight, toning and building muscle, becoming healthier, increasing your strength, recuperating from an injury, improving your balance, or finally having a six pack and the core strength to go with it. One goal we all have in common is that *we all want to succeed.*

More importantly, we all want to achieve our goals AS QUICKLY AS POSSIBLE! In the modern world, excelling and becoming successful is often dependent on doing something faster than the next guy. Many of us have the "the faster is better" mindset. The popular approach to fitness has become no different—our time spent working out needs to be used as efficiently as possible.

If we all work out because we want results, why would we limit ourselves to "exercising" while sitting down? This common resistance training approach is far from efficient.

A Fundamental Fitness Failure

The biggest problem in the fitness industry is seated exercise. Sitting down requires less energy, less muscle activity, and less coordination.

I've walked into fitness facilities and gyms all across America. All of them have sections of benches and machines. What do ALL of these machines and benches have in common? They all provide a comfortable place for you to sit on your ass!

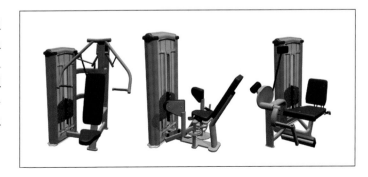

Compared to any form of locomotion, a seated position allows for a dramatic decrease in work from so many parts of the body. But because we are so accustomed to sitting, it has become part of everything we do, even "exercise."

Day after day, hours go by while we sit...

We sit down on our way to work,
We sit down for hours at work,
We sit at the gym.
We sit down for dinner, and we sit down through the evening before finally going to bed.

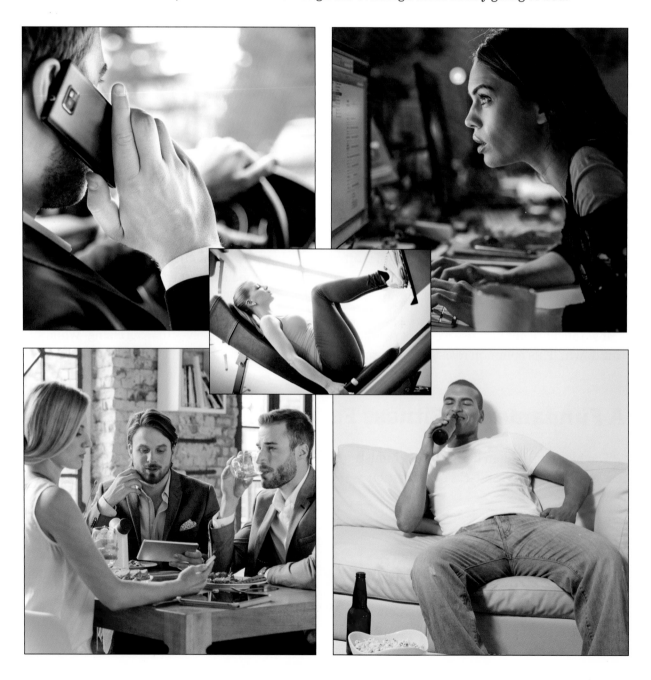

INTRINSIC STRENGTH TRAINING

People have become so accustomed to sitting that we have even developed "exercises" and machines to work each body part while sitting down. It sounds ridiculous, and we all know sitting is much easier than standing up—which is still much easier than changing foot positions while we exercise. Sitting should only be considered as a regression from standing upright or moving when designing your workouts.

Sitting for the majority of your workout will only limit your results. With our high calorie food intake and sedentary lifestyle, moving as much as possible should be the primary objective of a workout.

Less Energy Stimulates Less Muscle

Compared to sitting, standing upright and walking requires much more muscular activity. If bones are moving, then muscles are working. The amount of energy spent during one hour of an activity is known as its MET (Metabolic Equivalent of a Task). A single MET equals one calorie per hour, per kilogram of bodyweight. 1 MET = 1 kcal/kg/hr.[2] Walking (continuously stepping) will use 3.3 more METs on average as compared to sitting. For example, I currently weigh 200lb, so I would burn up to 90 more calories per hour if I were walking instead of sitting.[7,8,9]

Luckily, Intrinsic Strength Training® incorporates continuous steps into each exercise.

Electromyography (EMG) further demonstrates significantly less muscular activity throughout the legs in a seated position compared to standing and stepping. The study shown below examined the amount of voltage traveling through the legs while sitting, standing up, standing still, and stepping for the duration of a minute.

This electromyogram clearly indicates the lack of muscular activity while sitting.

Imagine how much energy (calories) you could burn while actively stepping during your resistance training. [3,4,5]

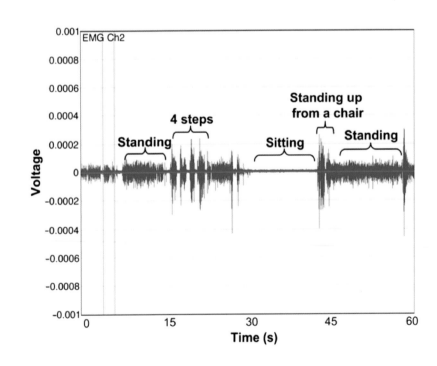

Seated bicep preacher curls, seated shoulder presses, seated rows, seated lat pull downs, seated leg extensions, seated dips, lying leg presses, lying chest press, lying skull crushers and lying hamstring curls are all perfect examples of exercises that supply the body with a great deal of assistance. All these conventional gym exercises disregard dynamic, full-body integration. In other words, conventional gym exercises disregard how our body is designed to operate as one interwoven structure.

Holding a weight while challenging the body to move is much more physically and mentally demanding than holding a weight in a seated position with the assistance of a chair. In all forms of locomotion, every muscle has to work together to balance and stabilize the body. This productive synergistic integration (6) of all the muscles and connective tissue is the key to a symmetrical, naturally shaped, healthy physique.

When we sit, the chair provides another point of contact for the body, making it much easier to balance and stabilize ourselves. The chair holds the pelvis still, limiting the amount of energy and muscular activity which could have come from using the 630+ muscles of the human body.

Sitting down while exercising is absolutely the laziest concept the fitness industry has ever adopted.

The practice of seated resistance training—with free weights or machines—needs to stop.

When lowering the body towards the ground during a lunge, there is consistent activity in every leg muscle, as well as the entire body.[11B] During a conventional leg exercise such as the seated leg extension machine, muscle activity is not consistent when compared to the standing lunge.

Muscles used during leg press

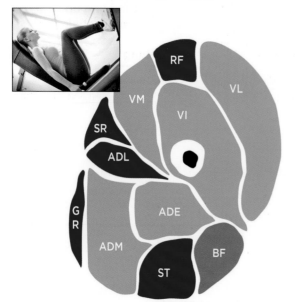

Muscles used during a seated machine knee extension

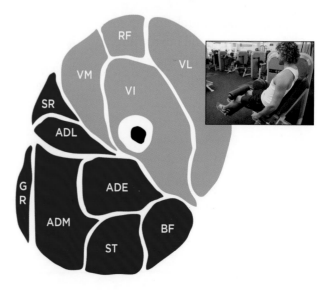

The referenced study shows that the real-world step squat activity will challenge the body much differently than an outdated approach which targets the same muscles but fails to simulate consistent muscle integration with the whole body. The artificial assistance from traditional machine-based exercise is a huge problem, because these machines will never replicate how the body works while standing up on two feet.

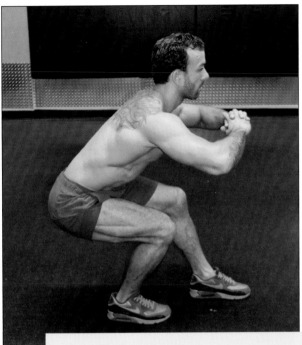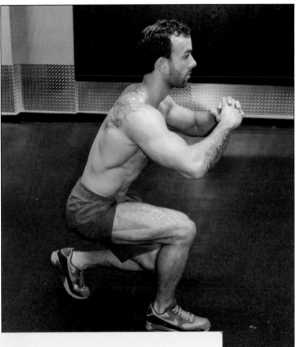

Notice how the rear and front step squat uses the many muscles of the entire leg together, as opposed to the leg press.

Over time, repeatedly challenging your body with the same seated exercises and machines in the same exact positions will only limit your full athletic potential. If we only train the body to be successful and strong on seated machines, the body will not be strong and successful in various upright positions.

If you are interested in getting more from your workout, skip the machines and avoid all seated exercises. Instead, focus on improving how well you can control your entire body during all of your workouts.

Each Intrinsic Strength Training® exercise simultaneously challenges your upper and lower extremities while localizing a specific muscle group. The dynamic unilateral resistance exercises of IST require more physical effort and mental concentration as compared to classic resistance training. Only through core integration can the muscles of the upper and lower extremities work in conjunction.

The more practice the body has moving, the better the body will move. Movement is LIFE. Each challenging physical task during a typical day will actively require simultaneous movement of the arms and legs while standing upright.

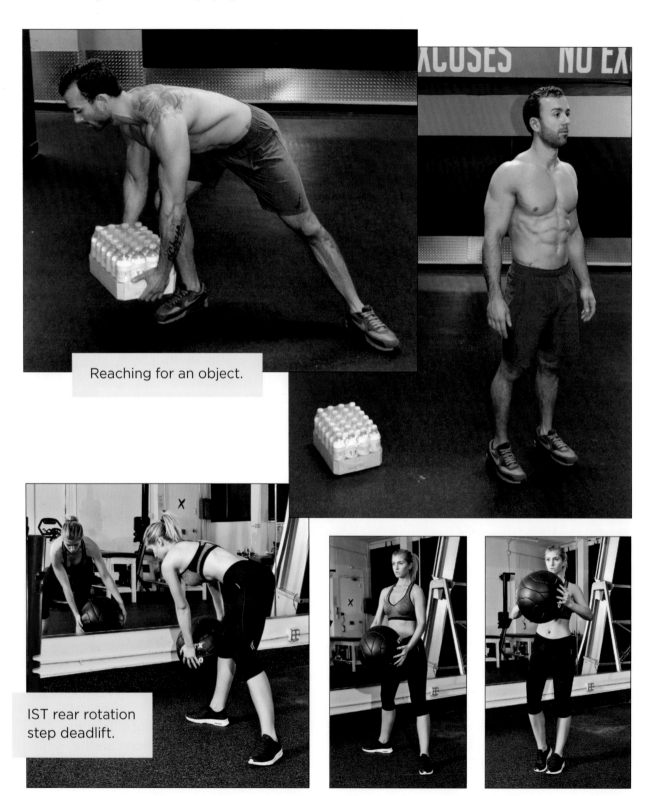

Reaching for an object.

IST rear rotation step deadlift.

INTRINSIC STRENGTH TRAINING

Why limit yourself to only building strength in static positions when you can be strong while moving through various upright positions. Rarely does any physically strenuous task outside the gym require you to stand perfectly still, sit down, or allow some muscles of the body to rest.

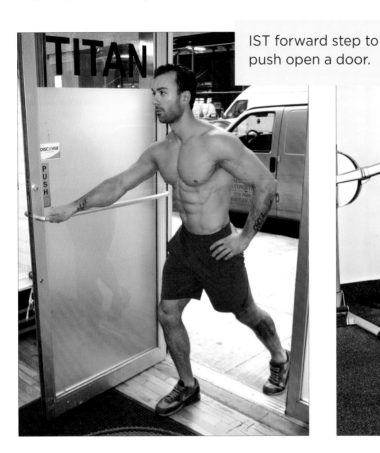

IST forward step to push open a door.

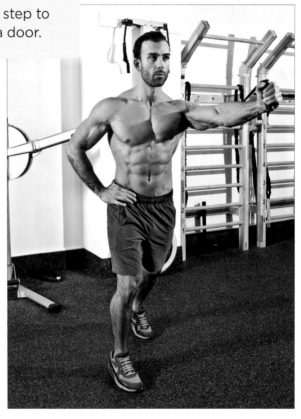

When you push open a heavy door, a chair does not magically pop up out of the wall, providing a place for you to sit during this task. Amazing physical feats are rarely accomplished in a seated position. Except for a few rare occasions, physically remarkable feats usually require the use of the entire body.

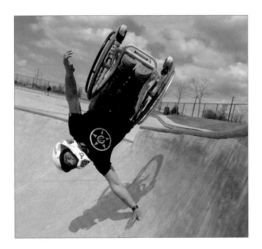

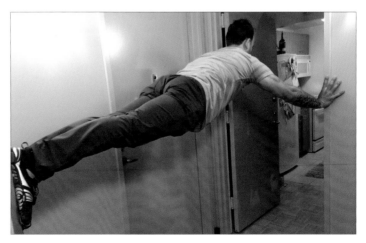

(1) Sophie B. P. Chargé, Michael A. Rudnicki (2004). "Cellular and Molecular Regulation of Muscle Regeneration". Physiological Reviews Jan 2004, 84 (1) 209-238; DOI: 10.1152/physrev.00019.2003

(2) Ainsworth, Barbara E.; Haskell, William L.; Herrmann, Stephen D.; Meckes, Nathanael; Bassett, David R.; Tudor-Locke, Catrine; Greer, Jennifer L.; Vezina, Jesse; Whitt-Glover, Melicia C.; Leon, Arthur S. (2011). "2011 Compendium of Physical Activities". Medicine & Science in Sports & Exercise 43 (8): 1575–81. doi:10.1249/MSS.0b013e31821ece12. PMID 21681120. https://sites.google.com/site/compendiumofphysicalactivities/corrected-mets

(3) http://www.juststand.org/Tools/CalorieBurnCalculator/tabid/637/language/en-US/Default.aspx

(4) http://www.livestrong.com/article/73916-calories-burned-standing-vs.-sitting/

(5) http://www.ehow.co.uk/about_5472437_calories-burned-standing-vs-sitting.html

(6) "synergistic." Collins English Dictionary – Complete and Unabridged. 1991, 1994, 1998, 2000, 2003. HarperCollins Publishers 22 Mar. 2015 http://www.thefreedictionary.com/synergistic

(7) http://www.ergotron.com/Portals/3/literature/compendium-of-physical-activities.pdf

(8) http://en.wikipedia.org/wiki/Metabolic_equivalent

(9) http://www.stillwater.k12.mn.us/sites/default/files/public/downloads/staff/JPAH%202012-1.pdf

(10) Dynamic Stability - http://adg.stanford.edu/aa241/stability/dynamicstability.html

(11) Tesch P A 1993 Muscle meets magnet. PA Tesch, Stockholm pg. 46, 47,59

(11B) Richardson, C., & Hodges, P. (2004). Therapeutic exercise for lumbopelvic stabilization a motor control approach for the treatment and prevention of low back pain (2nd ed.). Edinburgh: Churchill Livingstone.

LIFE

IS

NOT

STATIONARY

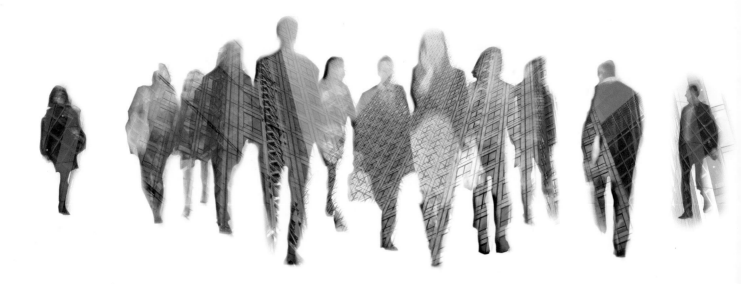

Throughout history, humans have often migrated thousands of miles on foot to survive. In many ways, not much has changed, we are still required to move from one place to another. We move our bodies from each location the very same way—one step at a time. Walking is our most common activity. Walking from place to place requires various continuous steps. So, why does our modern approach to exercise fail to challenge and train the body with various steps?

Throughout our lives, we will always be required to move. Resistance training needs to replicate how we move—one step at a time.

CHAPTER 4

Pieces Move Together to Move the Whole

With all forms of locomotion (moving from point A to point B) the entire body is required to work together. Stepping, walking, running, jumping, leaping, bounding, lunging, swimming, climbing, crawling, rolling, pushing and pulling all require the upper and lower extremities to work in unison as the position of the entire body changes throughout each form of locomotion.

If every part of the body is required to work together synergistically to replicate the most common forms of locomotion, why do most approaches to exercise and fitness training fail to replicate that synergy?

Visualize picking your laundry up off of the floor. As you walk over to pick up the laundry bag, did you take the time to step directly in front of the bag and then spend even more time to put your feet in a perfectly even bilateral stance before reaching for it? Most likely not, because that takes too much time, and this is not a 1RM (one rep max) effort deadlift.

While approaching the bag you most likely walked up to it without thinking, and simultaneously reached for it as you took your last step towards the bag.

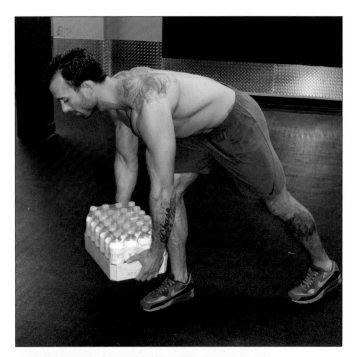

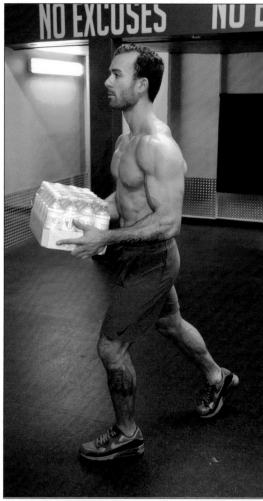

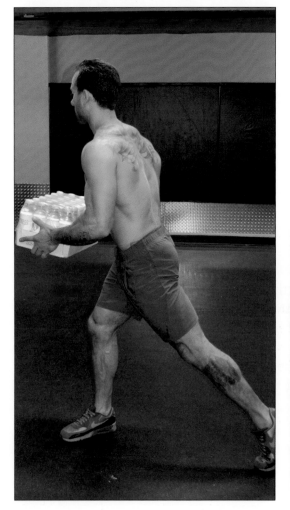

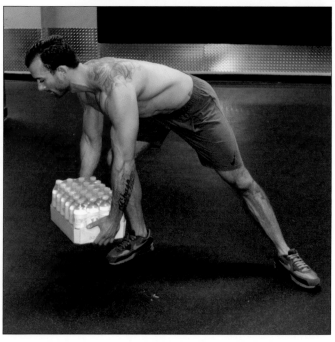

INTRINSIC STRENGTH TRAINING

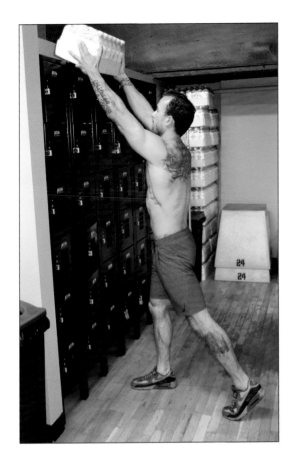

The lower extremities are often required to move simultaneously with the upper extremities. Rarely do our feet remaining stationary in a bilateral stance.

When carrying a box to its place on a high shelf, you are simultaneously required to lift the box while stepping closer to the shelf. This action requires a simultaneous lower extremity step with an upper extremity lift and reach.

Both of these physical tasks are only possible with simultaneous upper and lower extremity activity. All upright activity will require all of the body's muscles, connective tissue, and bones to move together. This undeniable fact can be observed during most common chores, hobbies and recreational activities.

In life, whenever we're challenged with a strenuous task, it's rare to have assistance from a seat or bench. It is also rare that we are required to stand entirely still, or focus on moving one particular muscle group while the rest of the body remains inactive.

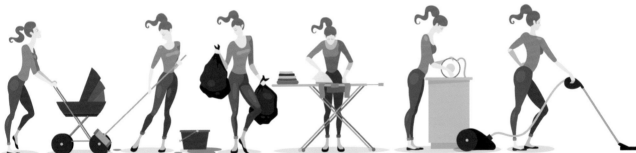

Consider the majority of general resistance training exercises and machines in a typical gym. Resistance training rarely—if ever—challenges the upper and lower extremities simultaneously. Often, we choose to exercise in a seated, assisted, and stationary position as a simple way to isolate a muscle group or to get a one rep max.

But, these exercise methods fail to challenge us in the same way the body moves throughout the day. Restricting movement to a perfect bilateral stance, lying on a bench, or leaning on a machine is a limited approach to exercise and will inhibit your body's full athletic potential.

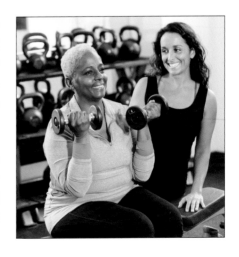

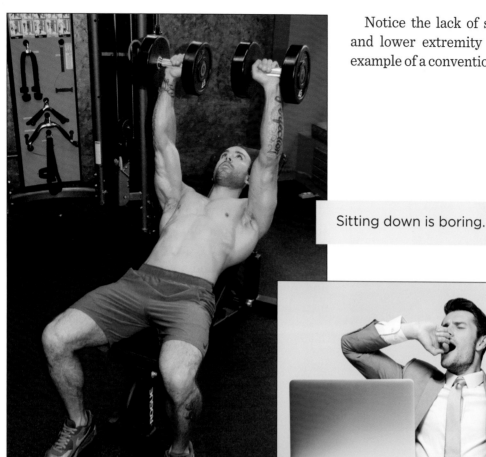

Notice the lack of simultaneous upper and lower extremity integration in this example of a conventional gym exercise.

Sitting down is boring.

Classic resistance training needs a makeover and should be approached with full body integration and locomotion in mind. Intrinsic Strength Training® will simultaneously challenge the upper and lower extremities by continually changing foot positions (stances) with every exercise.

The more time you spend training your entire body to move together, the better you will be at moving your entire body together.

If you felt more confident, able, and strong on your feet, how much different would your life be? Or, are you only interested in feeling confident, able, and strong while standing still and sitting down?

We Will Always Achieve More as a Whole

How well we can reach for something is dependent on how much of the body can be recruited to help. When we stand, every part of the body can help with the task at hand.

Seated vs. Standing Reach Test

1. Stand up with feet shoulder width apart.
2. Reach directly to your right—reach to an equal distance with BOTH arms.
3. Even though we consciously thought about moving just our arms, what else moved?
4. Notice how the entire body rotated toward the same side you were reaching—all the way down to your feet and ankles.
5. The body is designed to work as a whole, and to share the work. It equally distributed the task at hand to protect any single joint from being over-stressed or overworked.
6. Now, try this same task while sitting down.
7. Notice that it's virtually impossible to reach as far with your hands. Can you feel the limitation through your lower back?

When reaching with both hands directly to your right, you'll experience two different outcomes while sitting and standing. While sitting, the lower extremities are unable to assist the upper body in the reach. As the lower body remains at rest—with restricted movement—the upper body is required to handle the entire task. When part of the body's movement is restricted by sitting, it will be impossible to reach the same distance as compared to when standing.

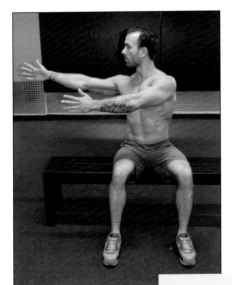 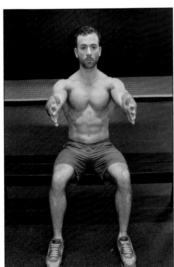 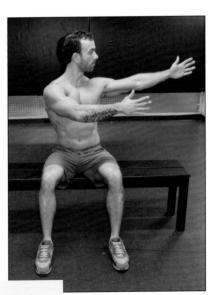

Hand position of side reach while seated...

Full body success can only occur when the entire body can efficiently distribute a task. Remember, every physical task will have a greater success rate with a whole body approach.

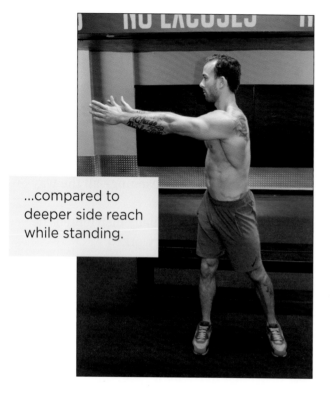

...compared to deeper side reach while standing.

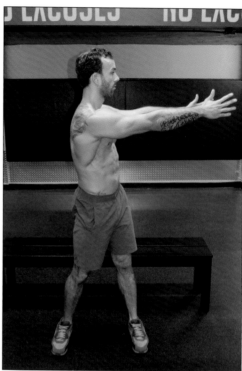

Now try these movements:

1. Stand with your feet shoulder width apart.
2. Put your left hand on your stomach to feel the musculature of your core.
3. Use your right hand to reach as far left and as far right as possible.
4. Notice how the core muscles engage as the movement of your arms and shoulders cause the entire body to move.

Can feel your abdominals engage as they react to the changing position of your shoulders?

As you reach to the side, look a little lower to notice that your legs and pelvis are no longer facing directly forward. The position of the legs and pelvis change as the shoulders' position changes while reaching. This process constantly requires the engagement of your core musculature.

CHAPTER 5

The Core Does More

Six pack abdominals are only the surface of the core. An amazing core brings more to the table than just looking awesome, a great core allows the body to be awesome!

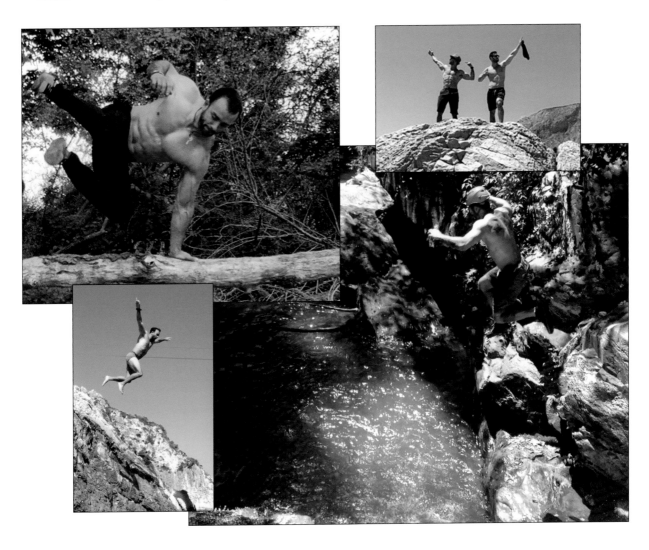

Connected to the Core

Was your home built on a strong and stable foundation made with solid bricks and cement? Or was your home built on soft, shifting sand? For a structure to stand tall and strong, it needs a stable foundation to distribute the multi-directional forces of mother nature.

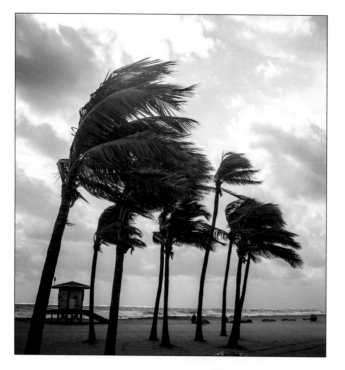

Although six pack abdominals look incredibly impressive, the role of abs in the human body is much greater than just aesthetics. Possessing an adequate core, with its multiple layers of muscle, enables you to combine the power of the upper and lower extremities into one integrated structure.

Imagine that your core is the foundation of your home, and your extremities are the walls and roof. A weak foundation will have adverse effects on a home's quality and longevity. Over time, a weak foundation will cause the walls to crack, the roof to leak, and the doors to creak. In time, as foundation repairs are neglected, the entire structure will change for the worse and may even begin to lean toward one side.

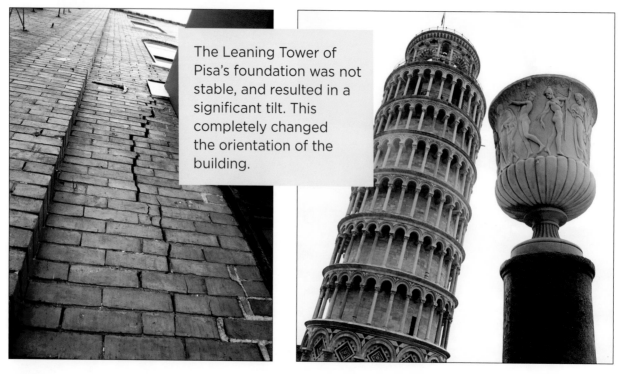

The Leaning Tower of Pisa's foundation was not stable, and resulted in a significant tilt. This completely changed the orientation of the building.

A weak foundation (core) will effect your structure (posture). Every structure has center of gravity, and our bodies are no different. The core shelters our vital organs, and it also provides a base for our extremities. The extremities and our entire torso (core) remain interconnected through layers of various types of connective tissue: ligaments, tendons, muscles, nerves, and fascia. Any time our extremities move while we are standing upright, they will always influence and activate the muscles of the core.

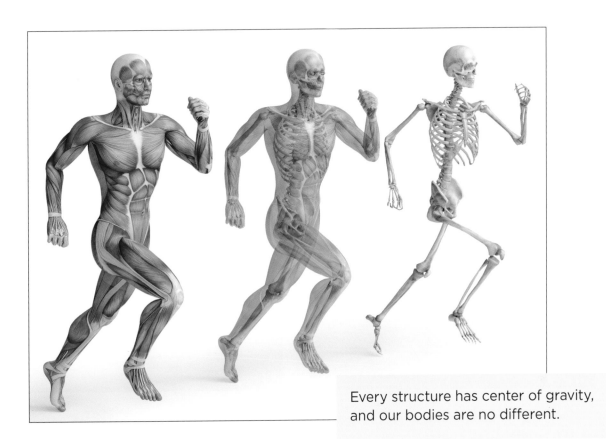

Every structure has center of gravity, and our bodies are no different.

As We Step...

When we are standing upright, taking a forward step with one leg will change the orientation of the pelvis (hip). The pelvis doesn't remain perfectly level. The entire position of the body changes as the leg moves forward. The motion of the pelvis directly effects and activates the core musculature.

Try these movements to observe this effect:

1. Stand with your feet shoulder width apart.
2. Look down at your pelvis, it should be facing in the same forward direction as your shoulders.
3. Take a forward step with your right foot.
4. Now look down at your pelvis again.
5. Notice how moving your right foot forward changed the orientation of your pelvis. The pelvis should have rotated to the left as compared to the orientation of the shoulders.

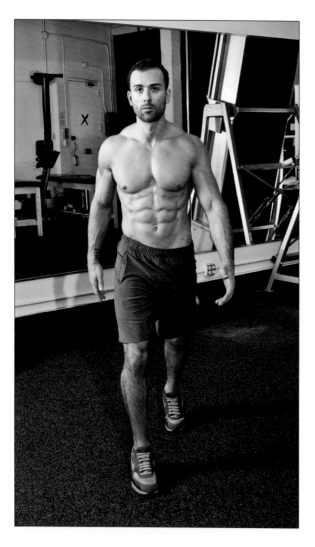
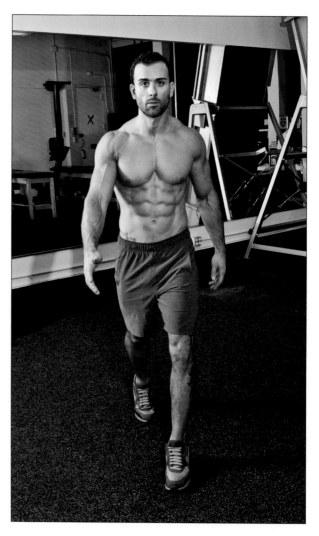

The pelvis remains connected to the lowest section of the spine (the lumbar/sacrum region) by the fusing of soft bone. The legs use multiple layers of connective tissue to remain interconnected with the pelvis and spine.

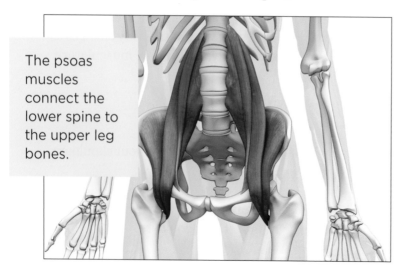

The psoas muscles connect the lower spine to the upper leg bones.

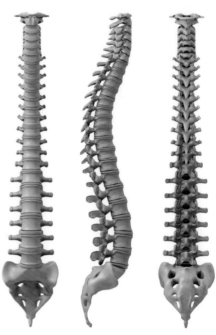

There is a direct correlation between the spine's position and the lower extremities—Moving the legs will directly affect the position and activation of the core's muscles.

Kicking is an example of how swinging a lower extremity creates tension in the core. This tension can be seen and felt through the abdominals.

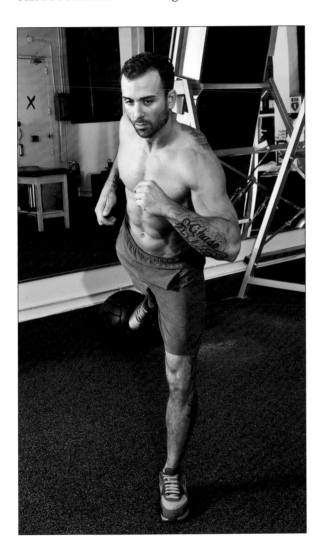 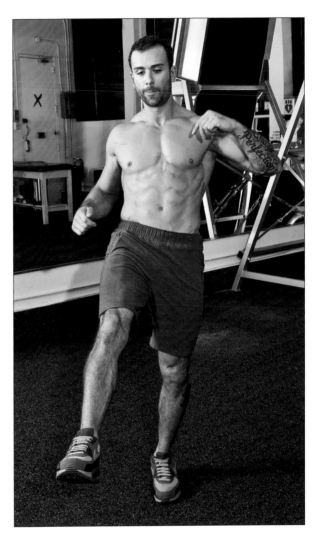

As We Reach...

When we are standing upright, reaching with either arm will change the orientation of the shoulder (scapula), affecting the position and activity of the core musculature.

Try this example:

1. Stand up straight while directly facing a mirror.
2. Reach your right hand across your body to the left, as far as possible.

3. Look into the mirror again.
4. How are your shoulders oriented?
5. Notice how your shoulders rotated toward the left as you reached left.

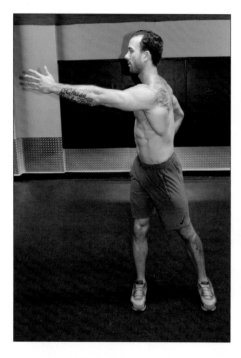 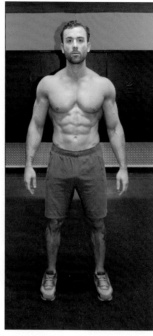 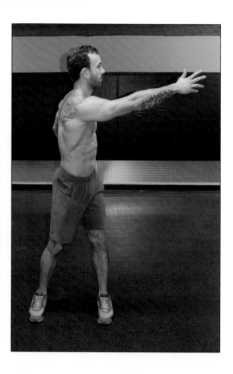

Our arms are bound to the upper torso by layers of connective tissue.

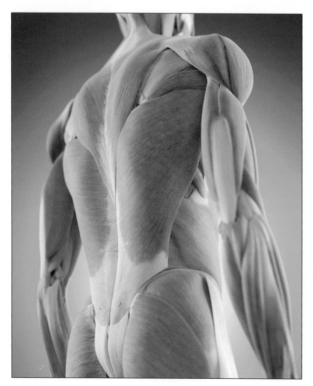 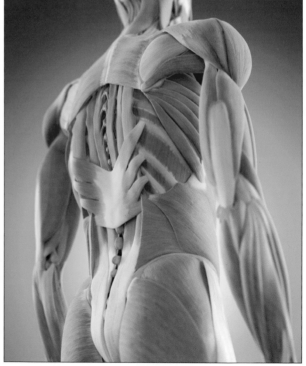

Throwing and punching are examples of how the upper extremities create tension which can be seen and felt through the abdominals.

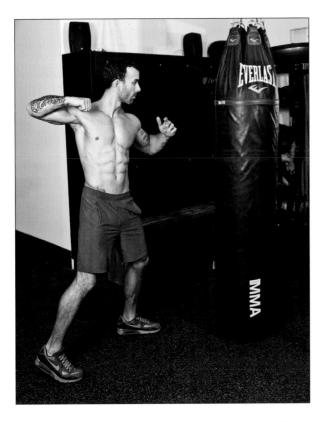
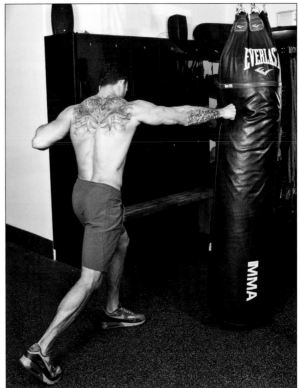

As We Walk...

Every step we take while walking also simultaneously causes the arms and legs to move, requiring constant and consistent core integration.

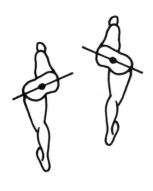

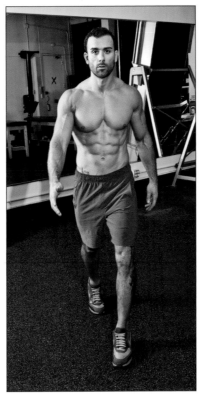
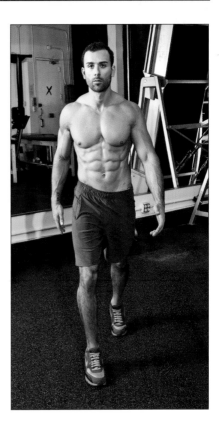

Our most natural and universal form of movement, walking, requires the simultaneous back and forth movement of the legs and arms, with a direct relationship to the rest of the body. The upper and lower extremities move in a reciprocal and simultaneous way—when the leg swings forward, the pelvis moves with it. When the arm swings forward, the shoulder position will change with it.[11]

After observing how the entire body moves as we reach, step, walk, kick and punch, we begin to understand that the consistent synergy between the upper and lower extremities is only possible through the integration of the core. The quality of this integration will determine how well we can control our bodies during all of our physical activities. The core is constantly required to react and control every motion from the arms and legs.

Full body integration is essential for providing balanced muscular tension throughout the body during any physical task. Being able to control compressive force from the body is just as important as reacting to—and distributing—compressive forces throughout the body.

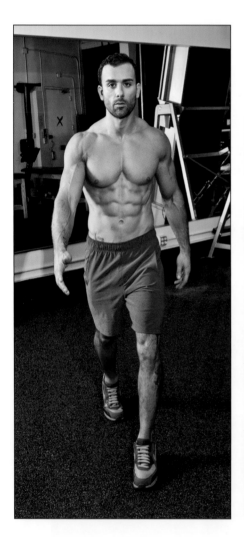
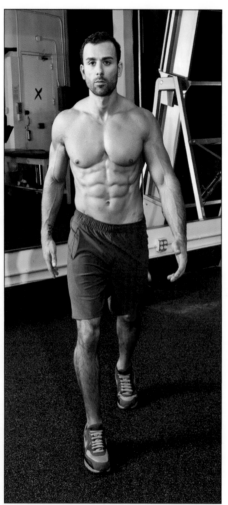

When the body is expected to slow down, restrict, or create any movement, all the connective tissue, muscles, bones, ligaments, and tendons contribute to the task at hand. This synergistic integration provides the essential and appropriate amount of tension needed to balance and stabilize the moving body.

The health and longevity of our joints is directly effected by how well the many pieces of the body can be controlled together while reacting to every possible position, speed, and internal or external force.

CHAPTER 6

Full Body Functions

As you now know, moving any of the extremities while standing upright will cause motion throughout the entire body.

A challenging task or activity will require the many segments of the body to integrate and work together synergistically. Our physical abilities and joint longevity depends on how well we can remain in control of the body's many parts. A healthy, athletic and efficient body will innately provide the correct amount of muscular tension needed to stabilize each joint. Whenever we initiate or stop any movement, intrinsic integration is essential. This integration is also an essential requirement for slowing down or moving an object.

When body control is subpar, the joints will suffer. Without the control necessary for a synergistic slowing down or speeding up of every body part, we can be assured of a lower rate of athletic success, and a higher risk of injury.

Slowing Down the Body and Sharing the Weight (Deceleration & Distribution)

Catching a falling object is a prime example of the body decelerating while simultaneously distributing the imposing force (the weight of the object) throughout the body.

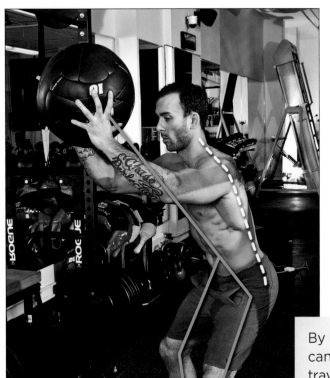

The "wall ball" exercise is a good example of deceleration and distribution in action. The exercise requires the segments of the body to work together when you catch the ball falling from overhead and slow it down before it slams you into the ground. Decelerating the force and weight of the ball while decelerating the weight and force of your body requires a lot of efficient muscle power. Generating the proper amount of tension needed throughout the body to do this safely requires efficient integration.

By standing, force can continue to travel into the ground through the legs.

The "wall ball" exercise would become extremely dangerous if it was possible to perform it while sitting down. When replicated in a seated position, the lower extremities are unable to assist with decelerating and distributing the force and weight of the body and the ball. Instead of the entire body sharing this workload, only the upper body would be able to contribute.

While sitting, the chair becomes the first contact point, and without the help of the lower extremities, the force and weight of the ball will be directed to the sit bones and lower back. The force would travel through the upper body towards the seat of the chair, causing the spine to suffer while in an extremely flexed position.

Excessive forces (heavy weight) can be dangerous and abusive to the spine while in a seated position. I would feel anxious about trying to catch a weighted object while sitting down. Catching something while standing is a different story. Standing allows the body to efficiently distribute the force of the propelled object evenly throughout the entire system.

Lifting while sitting down still loads the body with weight, but does not allow the entire body to distribute that weight.

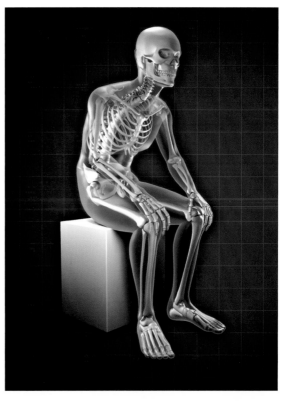

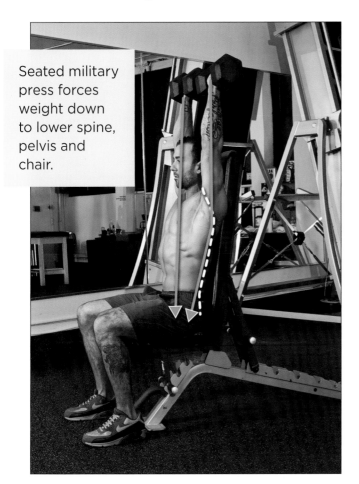

Seated military press forces weight down to lower spine, pelvis and chair.

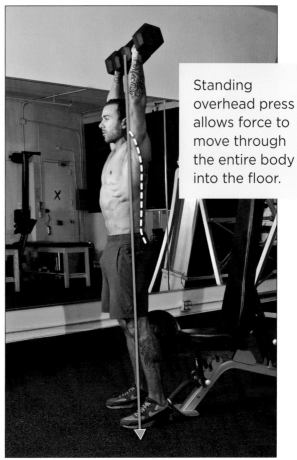

Standing overhead press allows force to move through the entire body into the floor.

Initiating Movement and Producing Force (Acceleration & Production)

Have you ever tried to punch something or someone while sitting?

If you have watched a heavy hitting boxer throw a punch, they produce the force for that punch with their entire body. If they were to punch from a seated position, their lower extremities would be unable to assist their upper extremities.

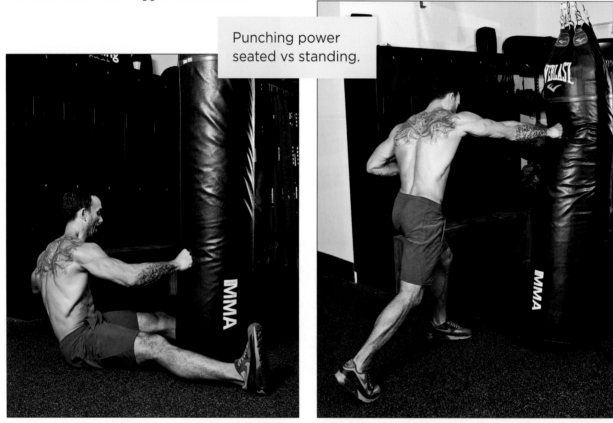

Punching power seated vs standing.

Clearly, the lower body can greatly assist the upper body when throwing a punch—and when the entire body contributes to the punch, it will be stronger and under control.

Similarly, our jumping ability and quality are directly effected by how well we can use our legs and arms to produce force together. Have you ever tried jumping while holding your arms still? Jumping without using the arms will limit the distance and height.

A max effort jump is a perfect example of producing force to accelerate the body. Try to jump up on something close to your max jump height. I am certain that you used your arms to help produce more explosive force. If you have tried jumping that high with your arms pinned to your sides, then you can clearly see how much the upper body assists in jumping.

Try this example:

1. Stand with an evenly spaced stance.
2. Keep your arms and hands relaxed by your sides.
3. Jump as high as you can without the assistance of your arms. It didn't feel very powerful, did it?
4. For the next jump, take advantage of the body's natural arm swing.
5. Notice that in a leg dominant activity, using your upper body makes a dramatic difference in the quality of the jump.

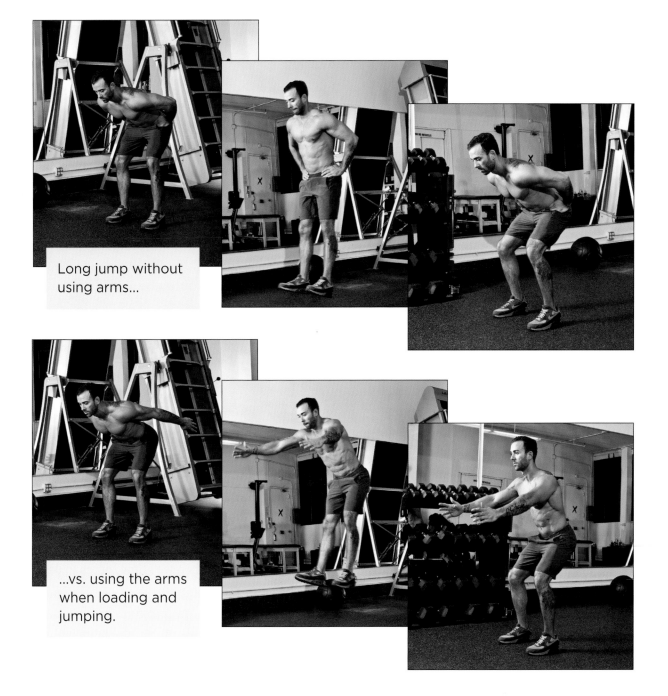

Long jump without using arms...

...vs. using the arms when loading and jumping.

Providing Full Body Tension Through Integration

Think of a long suspension bridge, such as California's Golden Gate. This bridge is designed to withstand an enormous amount of vehicle weight, forces of high-speed wind, and water current.

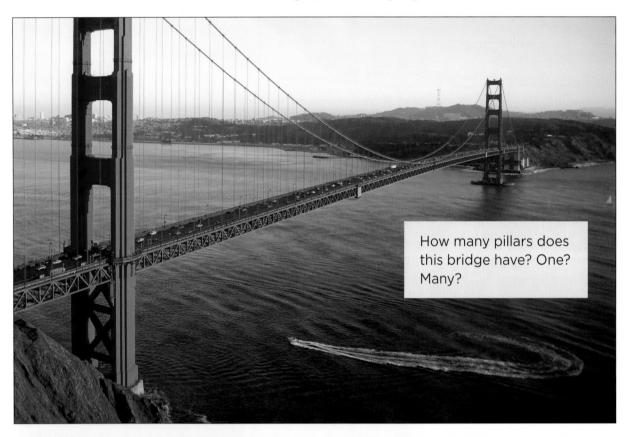

How many pillars does this bridge have? One? Many?

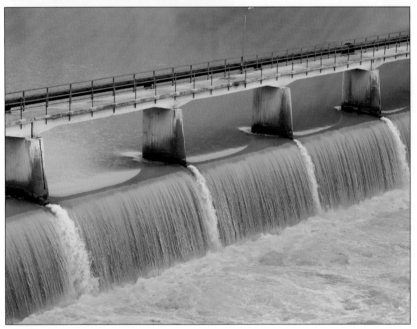

Instead of one thick, solid foundation that would dangerously restrict water flow, there are many separate support pillars under the bridge. Instead of fighting the force of the water's current, the pillars allow the forces to travel through the bridge. Like this bridge, our bodies are more successful when we allow forces to pass through instead of trying to stop these forces.

The bridge's interconnected suspension cables distribute tension throughout each section of the bridge, further increasing its weight handling capacity. Similarly, our bodies excel with a similar pillar and tension cable design. Our interconnected bodies resemble the design seen in Buckminster Fuller's structures of tensegrity.

A structure with tensegrity remains intact using a combination of tension and integrity. This interconnected dynamic structure can constantly adjust to the forces imposed on it without snapping in half or falling apart. A localized force will be distributed throughout an entire tensegrity structure as opposed to a localized force only affecting a localized area. [16, 17, 18, 19]

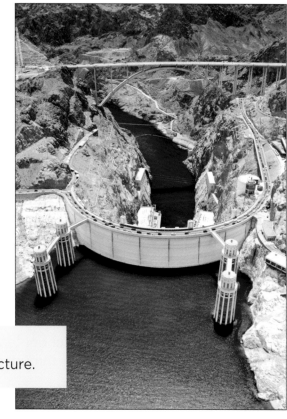

A localized force will be distributed throughout an entire tensegrity structure.

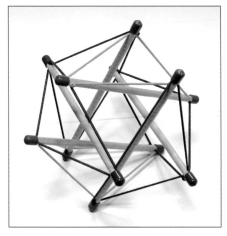

Multiple separate coil springs in a mattress make this possible.

The illustration below is an icosahedron, it is a tensegrity structure built with hard plastic and elastic strings. Notice how the structure can hold its shape without being completely solid. This lack of rigidity allows the structure to move and distribute each force imposed on it.

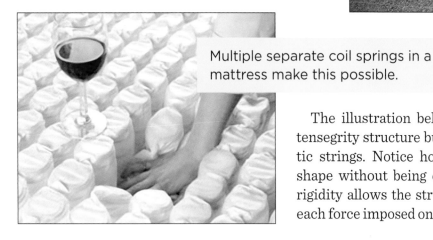

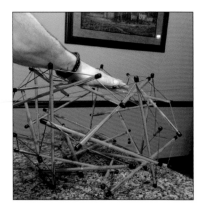

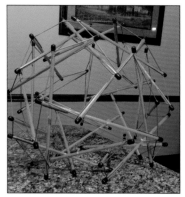

The bones throughout the body can resemble the hard pieces of plastic of an icosahedron. Likewise, our connective tissue, ligaments, tendons, fascia, muscles, skin, and nerves all replicate the elastic pieces of that same structure. Together, the ridged and elastic parts provide the appropriate amount of tension needed to distribute the forces traveling throughout the body.

The connective tissue which holds our structure together also allows our bodies to move freely when necessary. With connective tissue restriction, the body is able to react to each force imposed on it. When a force is removed, the body's structure will once again return to its original form. [16, 17, 18, 19]

> Together, the ridged and elastic parts of the body provide the appropriate amount of tension needed to distribute the forces traveling throughout the body.

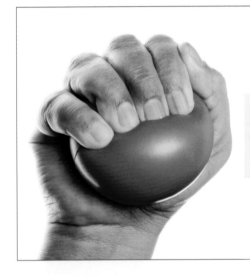

> When a ball is squeezed it compresses, but when the pressure is released, it comes back to its original form.

A Few Players Will Affect the Entire Team

Have you ever had an overly sore and tight muscle? Extremely sore muscles can inflict enough pain to throw off your natural groovement. Have you tried to walk down a stairwell after leg day?

One day after pushing myself through an extensive forefoot run, I woke up the next morning with super sore calves that completely effected the way I walked. While waddling down the street like a penguin, I realized that the range of motion in my feet was limited because of my overly tight and tender calves and restricted ankles. Walking symmetrically and gracefully was no longer an option.

The pain and stiffness associated with this muscular restriction caused a compensatory walking pattern. With excessive muscle tension, the foot and the ankle are unable to move freely, which will cause the entire body to move differently.

This principle holds true with any restricted muscles in our interwoven bodies. Whenever parts of the body are tight, restricted, weak or de-conditioned, the rest of the body must work overtime to compensate for them. These muscular imbalances and compensations directly effect your quality of life. They can also lead to poor posture, an asymmetrical physique, chronic pain, lack of balance, coordination, and confidence. Remaining in good health and maintaining physical symmetry is only achieved by understanding that the whole is greater than the sum of its parts.

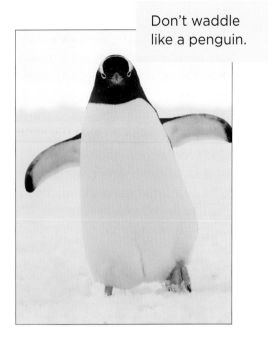

Don't waddle like a penguin.

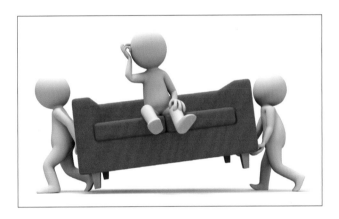

Have you ever had to move a couch with a few friends? There is always one friend who can barely hold up their end of the couch. (If you cannot relate, then you were probably the guy or gal that was struggling to hold up your end!) If one friend is not doing their fair share of work, then who and what does it effect? It effects the entire task (moving the couch) and it effects everyone involved. If one friend is unable to handle their share of the work, the other friends must overcompensate and pick up the remainder of the unsupported weight. The weight of the couch is no longer equally distributed between everyone. As you begin to drop your side of the couch to the ground, everyone else experiences much greater stress while trying to hold up their end.

Now, imagine this scenario as it happens inside the body—no matter the task, if one part of the body is unable to contribute to the task at hand, the other parts of the body have to over compensate for those lagging body parts.

Our Physical Success Relies on How Well We Can Distribute Force

How does a palm tree survive hurricane winds? It bends to distribute the extreme forces. A palm tree remains rigid enough to support its natural upright shape and fronds without bending. When extreme external forces such as hurricane winds are present, the tree will bend and sway to distribute the force of each gust. When the wind stops, the tree returns back to its original, upright position.

If the tree had a rigid structure that did not allow for any movement (bending), it would not be as successful in distributing the excessive force of the wind. When a structure is too rigid to move, its pieces will break apart when an external force becomes too intense.

If every bone in the human skeleton was fused together, or if all of the connective tissues were too tight to move, how well could our bodies distribute the force from a hard push to the shoulder?

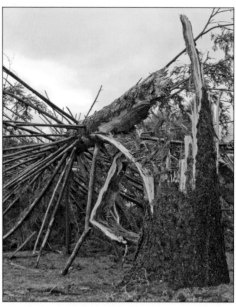

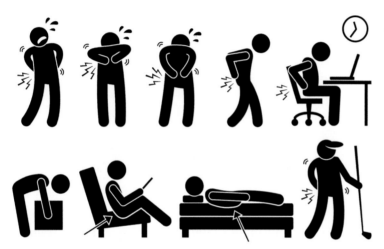

If every part of the body was unable to move when pushed, distributing those forces throughout the entire system would be impossible.

When an external force—such as someone trying to push you over—is imposed on the body, it must react. The appropriate amount of muscular tension throughout the body is essential to safely distributing this external force. Every physical activity requires the body to move, bend, rotate, and absorb external forces—how else would you survive?

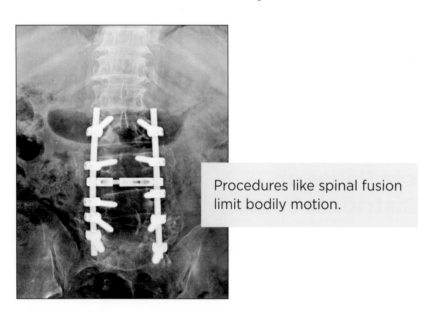

Procedures like spinal fusion limit bodily motion.

The human body has 206 bones, and is articulated through 230 joints within the structure of the skeleton, allowing for a lot of movement potential.

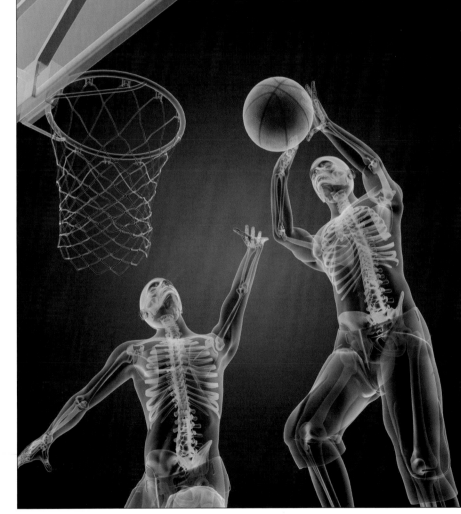

When we rotate, bend, and move, a substantial amount of motion is distributed throughout the entire body. Consider the corkscrew-like motion required of the spine when we rotate while reaching overhead and behind. Every joint within the extremities and the core—including the spine—must also rotate and extend.

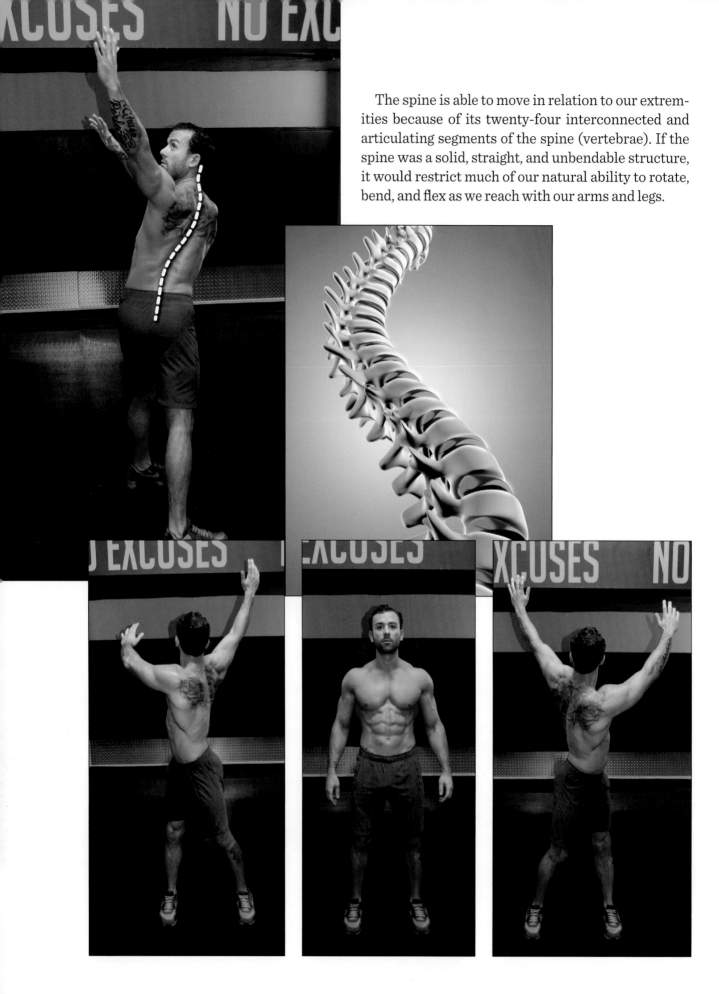

The spine is able to move in relation to our extremities because of its twenty-four interconnected and articulating segments of the spine (vertebrae). If the spine was a solid, straight, and unbendable structure, it would restrict much of our natural ability to rotate, bend, and flex as we reach with our arms and legs.

INTRINSIC STRENGTH TRAINING

For example, when we bend to the side (laterally), this doesn't result in a 90-degree bend in the middle of our bodies.

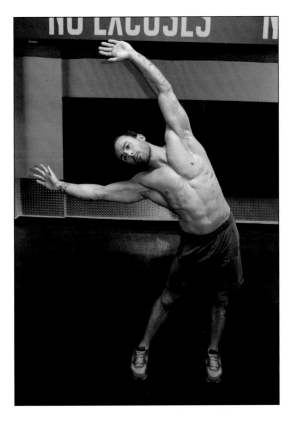
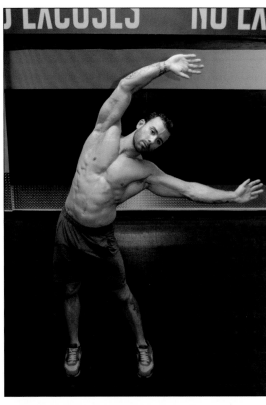
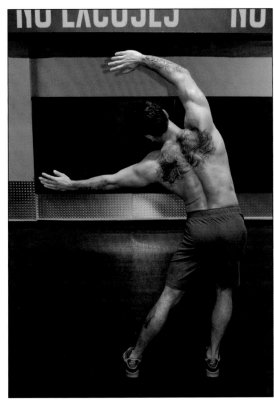
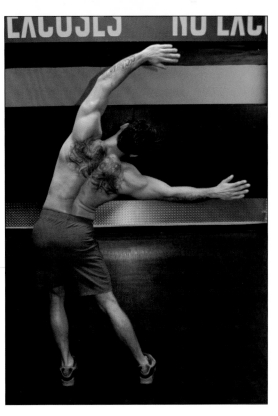

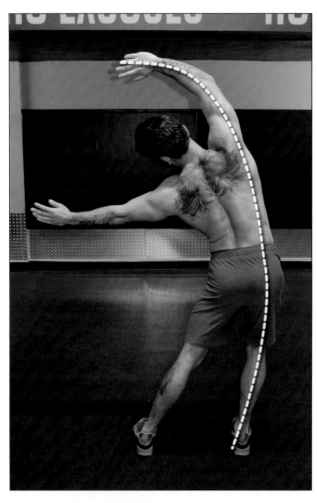

Notice how every joint in the body works together to create a full and smooth side bend. Each joint segment contributes a few degrees to the bend, though some joints will move more than others. When each joint can move without restriction, the body creates a safe and equally balanced lateral bend. This type of distributed full body motion through efficient joint integration is necessary for every upright activity.

The health and resilience of our connective tissue determines how all our joints move, and how well they are controlled. Your lifestyle, general health, approach to exercise, prior injuries, current mental stress level and hydration all contribute to the quality of your connective tissue. The state of all of the body's connective tissue directly effects the body's athletic abilities.

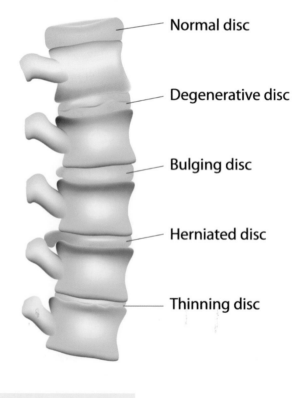

- Normal disc
- Degenerative disc
- Bulging disc
- Herniated disc
- Thinning disc

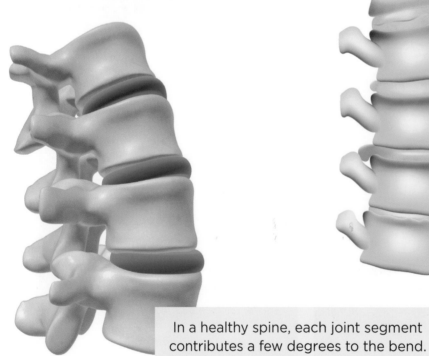

In a healthy spine, each joint segment contributes a few degrees to the bend.

CHAPTER 7

Protecting the Body from the Inside Out

Extensive periods of sitting are also extensive periods of muscular inactivity. Over time, less muscular activity degrades the high level of core conditioning you once had as a fearless and joyous child. Extensive periods of inactivity result in less blood and nutrients flowing to the muscles, ligaments, tendons, fascia, and joints, leaving them in a malnourished, weakened state.

In any physical activity, efficient core function is necessary for proper joint alignment as you move. Only well-integrated body parts can provide the appropriate muscle tension needed as we move. By learning to improve your body control, you will have more opportunities for meaningful life experiences and greater joy throughout your day.

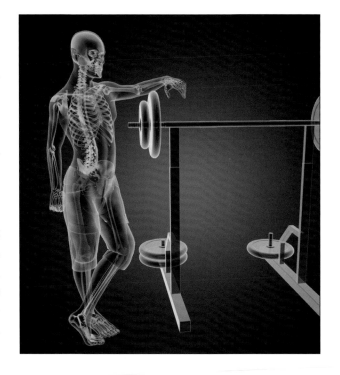

The core is required to react, control and stabilize every movement made by the upper and lower extremities. A less conditioned core leads to a weaker body, directly limiting your physical abilities and life experiences. Creating a foundation for the extremities and powerful, aesthetic muscles to move as needed is only possible through successful full body integration.

Intrinsic Strength Training® requires full body integration and a stable foundation. IST challenges your body to produce the appropriate amount of muscle tension through the core and the entire body to successfully complete every exercise. The combination of consistent dynamic stepping patterns and resistance training using in IST will improve how well your body can integrate itself as one unit. Challenging the body's abilities to integrate will improve your muscle control and joint alignment, prolonging your physical abilities.

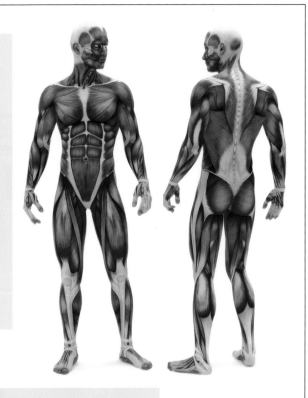

Intrinsic Strength Training® challenges the body with resistance while moving through different upright positions. This training strategy challenges the body to successfully apply tonic core tension. Tonic core tension is a natural and constant tautness of the core's multiple layers. These core muscles integrate into the other muscles of the body connected to the extremities.

Creating and improving the foundation can only be achieved by continually training the body as one dynamic, integrated unit. Upright resistance training improves muscular function by strengthening the extremities while integrating the core. [12, 20, 21]

Creating consistent core tension between the multiple layers of muscle is essential to the positioning of the body's joints.

This constant core tension is known as the body's "corset reaction". This reaction provides tonic (continuous) tension within the many interwoven parts of the core, directly controlling and stabilizing the individual segments of the spine and pelvis. This constant tension is needed when reacting to every move of our extremities and is essential to a healthy spine.

When Too Much is Too Much

Sometimes we demand too much from our bodies. A weight might be too heavy for an unstable core to withstand. It is difficult for an unstable core to safely distribute force throughout the body.

Bracing will always help the body handle an excessive load or any powerful force that requires maximum effort. Bracing the abdominals also ensures proper joint alignment through the hips and spine to provide core stability. Bracing the core is widely practiced for maximum effort, explosive activities such as powerlifting, martial arts, and extreme calisthenics. It is also one of our many natural defense mechanisms. When you are startled, your body immediately braces the core for protection, and to prepare for an expected force or impact.

Contracting the entire core as hard as you can while in an upright position will stimulate multiple layers of the core: the transverse abdominis, internal and external obliques, spinal erectors, psoas, and powerful gluteal muscles.

Tested and Proven.

You can produce greater maximum force while bracing your body. I performed a max grip test with a dynamometer to test this theory and compare muscle contractions while changing body positions.

I compared the maximum force of my grip while in the following positions: bilateral relaxed sitting, bilateral relaxed standing, bilateral standing while bracing, and split leg standing while bracing. The results show the amount of force (pressure in pounds) I was able to produce while squeezing the dynamometer with my right hand.

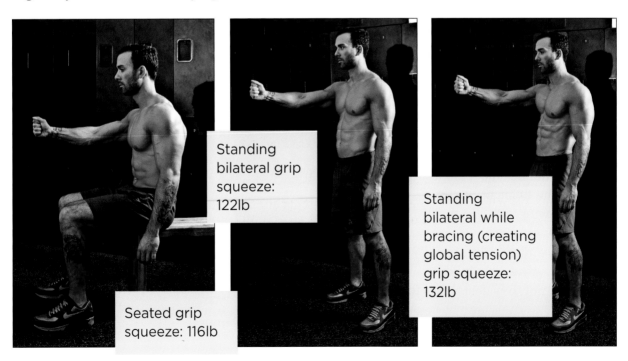

Standing bilateral grip squeeze: 122lb

Seated grip squeeze: 116lb

Standing bilateral while bracing (creating global tension) grip squeeze: 132lb

I was able to produce more grip force when more muscles were integrated with my efforts while bracing!

Please note that bracing does not require sucking in or sticking out your belly. Bracing is simply squeezing the entire core—abdominals and glutes—to create more tension throughout the entire body.[13] Bracing is essential for distributing excessive force (heavy loads, hard impacts, or uncertain situations) while maintaining safe and proper joint alignment.

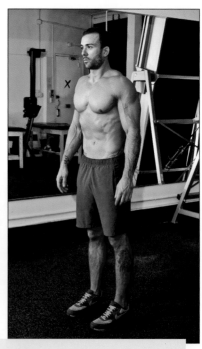

Standing split leg while bracing grip squeeze: 136lb

We Are NOT Hollow

Please note that when I refer to the "corset reaction" and bracing, I AM NOT referring to "hollowing" the core. Hollowing is a cue to suck in the stomach during an exercise in the attempt to improve core tension. However, this action will not increase the strength of your body. "Draw your navel to your spine" is a phrase commonly used in Pilates. This concept will increase the stimulation in only *one* muscle of the core, the transverse abdominis.[13]

Unfortunately, the action of "hollowing" will result in a less active, less stable core.[13] With less activity from other abdominal muscles like the internal and external obliques, this less active core will also lead to an overall weaker body during dynamic movement. Creating the habit of continually hollowing the core will essentially create a weaker body. Remember, abnormal actions during strenuous activity are not the safest things to practice.

Bracing (left) is simply squeezing the entire core—abdominals and glutes. "Hollowing" (right) will result in a less active, less stable core.

More Power with More Integration: Irradiation

As the entire body becomes integrated, it gains an amazing ability to produce more strength. The popular slogans, "There is no I in TEAM" and "Together we stand, divided we fall" are also true when describing how the human body works. As the body is challenged, the hardest working muscles will recruit their neighboring muscles.

When we struggle to accomplish a strenuous task and start to strain, our muscles will contract and tense even harder, producing more muscular force. This process, irradiation, is here to rescue us. The concept of irradiation is based on the idea that the human body is stronger when used as a whole. Increasing our strength for a maximum effort lift or activity is possible through global (full body) muscular contractions. Bracing the core and contracting all of the muscles throughout the body will cause an irradiation effect over the entire body, increasing the ability to complete the task at hand.

"The concept of irradiation is a physical rehabilitation technique that has its roots in PNF (proprioceptive neuromuscular facilitation). Simply put, the generation of a strong muscle contraction can directly increase the firing of weaker muscle groups that produce or assist with the desired movement pattern. Keep in mind that adequate trunk mobility and stability are prerequisites for optimal irradiation to the extremities." —Jeremy Baber, PT Founder of Rekinetics™

Neurons That Fire Together Wire Together

Muscles are connected and communicate through fascia, a fibrous net of connective tissue (made of collagen) underneath our skin which encapsulates every part of the body from head to toe. It intertwines every cell in our bones, muscles, ligaments, tendons, nerves, blood vessels and organs.[14]

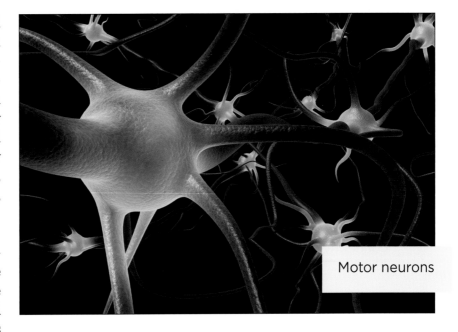

Motor neurons

All of the connective tissue within the body has the ability to send and receive information via electrical signals about sensations and motion through sensory and motor nerves. The proprioceptors throughout these tissues can distinguish the motion, location, and amount of compression of all the joints, as well as the amount

All of this proprioceptive information is relayed to the central nervous system (CNS) residing in the brain and spinal cord. The CNS enables the proprioceptors to evaluate, understand and control every position and sensation within the body. The CNS also controls how much tension the muscles and connective tissues can provide in every position of every activity.

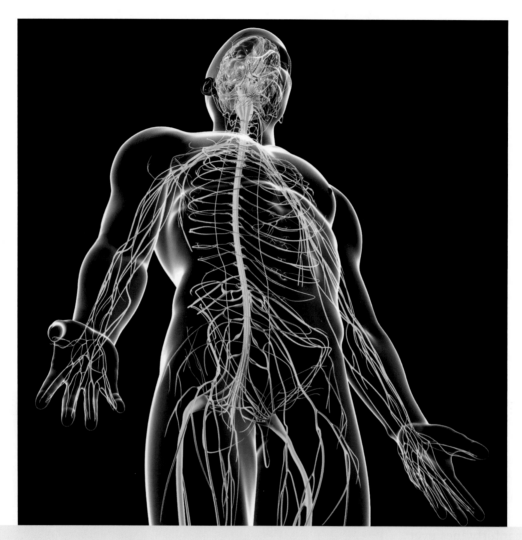

The full body tension created with every Intrinsic Strength Training® exercise promotes an irradiation effect throughout the entire body. Successfully controlling every joint as the body is dynamically challenged is only possible through the integration of all of the muscles and connective tissue.

CHAPTER 8

Walking
with Force

Every step we take transfers force throughout the body. We experience and benefit from these reactive forces with every step and every object we touch throughout the day. When our feet come in contact with the ground, the force of our weight and momentum is transferred to the ground. This transfer of force from one object (a foot) to another (the ground) is known as a contact force.

Newton's Third Law of Motion states that for every action, there is always an equal and opposite reaction. So, when two moving objects come into contact, there is a simultaneous exchange (transfer) of force from both objects. When the foot comes in contact with the ground, the foot's force is transferred into the ground. At the same time, a reactive force will be transferred back to the foot and throughout the body. [15]

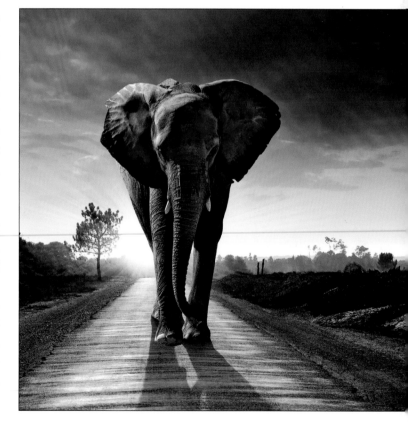

Newton's Pendulum is a great example of how energy is transferred through the contact of two objects. Notice what happens when the ball in motion contacts the motionless balls. The weight and momentum of the moving ball creates a force that is transferred to the motionless balls when contacted. The energy of the moving ball is transferred through the entire row of motionless balls until it finally propels the last ball outward.

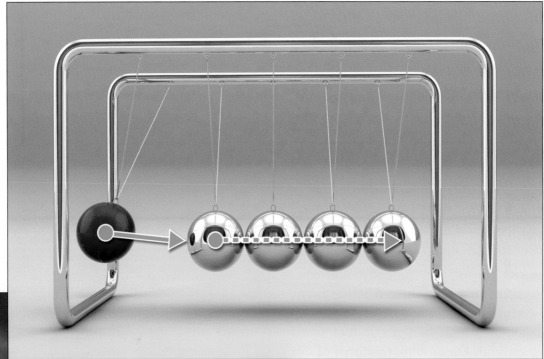

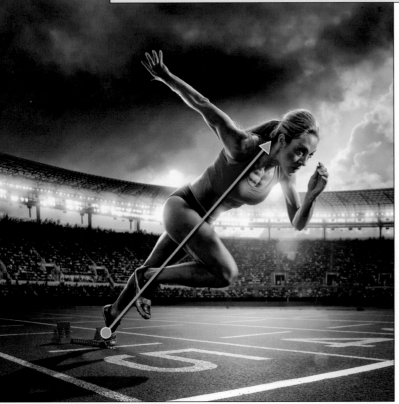

The same amount of force will continually transfer through the balls because there is no loss of force during this interaction. Without a loss of force, this transfer will continue back and forth until something inhibits it.

This is the same type of reactive force as when we step on the ground.

As gravity and momentum push our weight into the ground, the contact force produced from our feet hitting the ground will cause a reactive force to be transferred back into the foot. This force will then travel through the foot, up the leg and into the core. A forceful contact (action) will cause a forceful reaction known as ground reaction force (GRF).

Variables of Ground Reaction Force

The best surface for performing a task depends on the demands of the activity. When I want to run a 5k for my fastest time, I will choose to run on concrete or asphalt rather than a sandy trail. My running stride is much more efficient on a solid, paved surface compared to soft sand. Each stride on pavement provides an excellent ground reaction force to help propel my body with each step.

But sometimes I prefer a surface that can absorb the forces of my weight and momentum. When learning how to do a backflip or any aerial trick, I prefer sand, a gymnastics mat or a trampoline. These surfaces can all absorb some of the force of my weight and momentum. When learning, falling is inevitable and I would like to avoid pain or injury. I'm instantly grateful for those soft surfaces when they absorb my body's impact. As the soft surface absorbs some of my contact force, less reactive force will transfer back into my body.

Wasting Energy

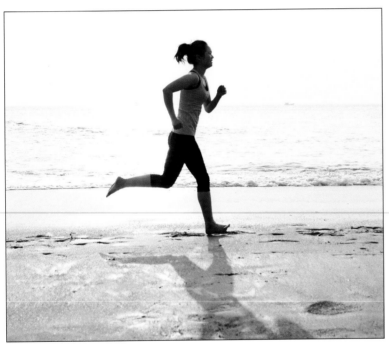

Have you ever tried walking in the sand? Each time your foot comes in contact with the sand, it sinks in and slides. When you step on a hard surface like concrete, the foot is unable to sink or slide into it. On any hard surface, like pavement, a normal walking pace is about three to four miles per hour. Have you ever tried walking at that pace in the sand? It's much more difficult than walking on the pavement. Walking in the sand immediately increases the required effort, and the heart rate elevates as the muscles are required to produce more force. As the foot comes in contact with—and sinks into the sand—the force is absorbed by the sand. Since the sand absorbs a lot of this force, this also reduces the reaction force, limiting how well each step can propel the body.

Ground reaction force effects how much effort is required for a task. When our energy is lost in the sand, the body must compensate with greater effort. This is why it's much more physically demanding to walk in sand than on pavement. Think about a car spinning its wheels in the sand. I'm still burning gas, but not moving. It is wasting energy.

Reaction forces travel through the entire body, not just the feet.

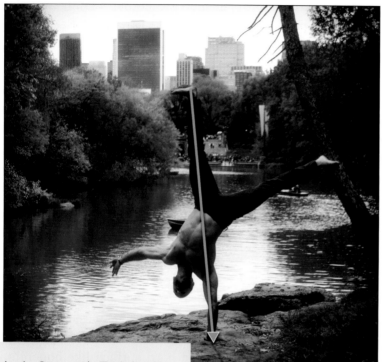

Since reactive forces travel through the entire body, learning to integrate and control the body is essential. *Learning enough control to distribute these omni-directional reactive forces is crucial for maintaining safe joint alignment through various positions. Sufficient body control, strength, and mobility is a critical factor for maintaining the safety and longevity of your body over time.*

Fortunately, the quality and success of maintaining control of your body improves with more practice.

Intrinsic Strength Training®'s dynamic and upright approach to resistance training will provide the body with the experience of omni-directional reactive forces through omni-directional body positions. As IST continually challenges the body to move with and against added resistance, all of the body's muscles and connective tissues will be forced to integrate for physical success. IST will better prepare you to take part in more physical activities with more confidence in your abilities, a key factor for living a full and satisfying life.

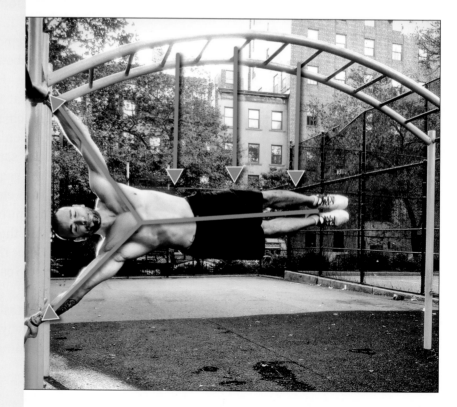

Do You Leak?

When beginning Intrinsic Strength Training®, some exercises may challenge you more than others. Controlling your extremities well enough to maintain efficient balance and control is essential to the success of each exercise, so take the time to learn how to create the appropriate amount of muscle tension and mobility needed throughout the body.

Sometimes the amount of force imposed on our bodies is too much to manage. So, if a weight is too heavy and you are unable to maintain a safe body position and joint alignment while applying proper core tension, please re-center yourself and reduce the resistance load. When the muscles and connective tissue fail to control the body, the joints will suffer. Our joints are not indestructible, they are made of connective tissue (joint capsule, ligament or cartilage) and are responsible for connecting all of our 206 bones. We have joints that pivot, slide, swivel, rotate, and hinge. Where ever there are moving parts, there will be friction between them, and friction causes wear and tear.

A joint will degenerate faster when your body is unable to control the forces imposed on it. With less body control, there's a higher probability of failure during a physical task—along with a greater risk of muscular or skeletal injury. Many factors effect joint wear. How much do you move every day? How does your posture look? Do you spend hours sitting in a slouched position with your face down while looking at your computer or phone screen? Do your gym workouts involve even more sitting? Does your physical activity amount to less than seven hours a week? Do you consume processed foods? Do you drink less than your suggested daily water intake?

If you have answered yes to these those questions, then you probably do not have a rock solid core that can effortlessly maintain a symmetrical and assertive posture while moving throughout the day. We should both agree that some changes are necessary. Fortunately, learning to control and use the body as one integrated unit will reduce joint tissue friction—and wear and tear.

When beginning Intrinsic Strength Training®, some exercises may challenge you more than others. Controlling your extremities well enough to maintain efficient balance and control is essential to the success of each exercise, so take the time to learn how to create the appropriate amount of muscle tension and mobility needed throughout the body.

The many joints and muscles of the body can create a LOT of movement, but how well can you control it?

A lot of movement—but without body control is like a race car with a bad driver. All the potential for amazing performance, speed, and ability is there, but cannot happen without the driver. Instead of smoothly rounding each corner under control, a bad driver with poor car control will always swerve, slide and brake incorrectly.

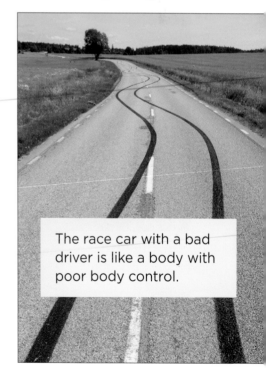

The race car with a bad driver is like a body with poor body control.

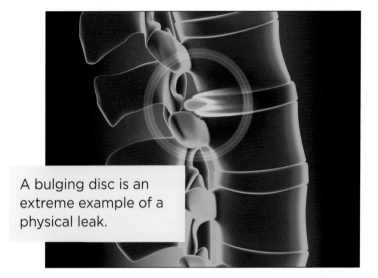

A bulging disc is an extreme example of a physical leak.

These inefficiencies also cause rapid wear and tear on the tires and brakes which are expensive to replace—just like hips and knees.

The race car with a bad driver is like a body with poor body control. Our joints wear down from energy leaks just as the race car's brakes and tires are destroyed by an inexperienced driver. All parts of a perfectly trained body work together to equally and efficiently distribute the forces of every physical task.

Energy leaks are more likely to occur within a weaker, restricted and uncoordinated body. When we fail to efficiently distribute force throughout our entire bodies, our physical abilities and chances of physical success are considerably limited.

Energy leaks effect the body in a similar way as slipping in sand. When a foot transfers force into the sand, the force is absorbed by the moving sand. Similarly, when a force is transferred through the joints of the body, and moves an unstable joint, the force is absorbed by that joint.

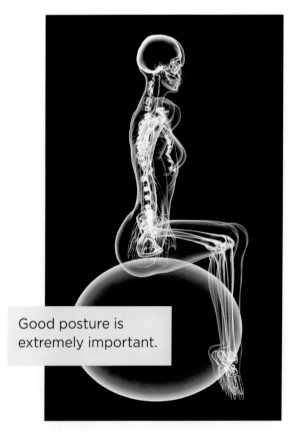

Good posture is extremely important.

With proper training, we can learn successful, full-body integration in any position. Equal distribution of a workload through all of our connective tissue is essential for proper joint alignment as we move. As a force's location, type, amount, and speed changes, the body must have enough mobility and instantly generate just enough tension to withstand that force. The body must remain passive enough to fluidly distribute these forces while still moving freely. With proper alignment, distributing and producing the forces needed to participate in strenuous activities is much easier and much more efficient.

If your approach to exercise lacks full body dynamic integration, life's external stressors will gradually but negatively impact your physique, posture, and lifestyle. A sedentary lifestyle and a seated, stationary approach to fitness creates asymmetries and areas of weakness. Inefficient areas of weakness cause more energy leaks and postural compensations. Disruption of the body's natural unity causes surrounding areas to work harder, become overly tight, and restrict the motion of the spine, hips, shoulders, and extremities. As muscular and postural asymmetries form and build over time, even an average person will notice your poor posture. Good posture is extremely important as it directly affects how we are perceived by others.

As symmetry is lost, our natural ability to move freely and efficiently is greatly compromised. Maintaining safe body positions while reacting to the unexpected forces of life becomes much more difficult without proper body control.

So ask yourself, do you want to leak?

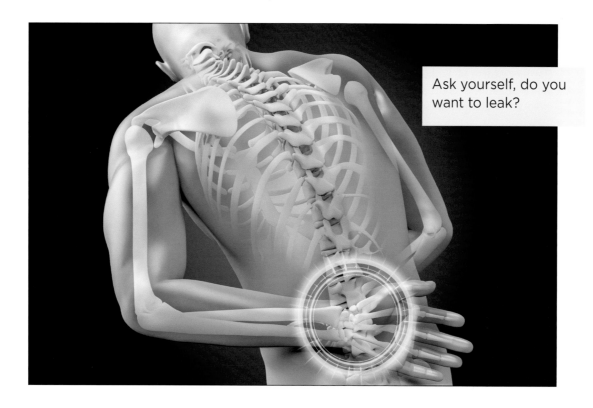

(12)   The Gray Institute

(13)   Danneels L A, van der Straeten G G, Cambier D C, Witvrouw E E, Cuyper H J 2000 CT imaging of tnUlk muscles in chronic low back pain patients and healthy control subjects. European Spine Journal 9:266-272

(14)   McGill, Stuart. Low Back Disorders: Evidence-based Prevention and Rehabilitation. 2nd ed. Champaign, IL: Human Kinetics, 2007. 171-176. Print.

(15   Clinical Application of Neuromuscular Techniques: The upper bod By Leon Chaitow, Judith DeLany pg 1-5

(16)   http://en.wikipedia.org/wiki/Newton%27s_laws_of_motion#Newton.27s_third_law

(17)   A Fuller Explanation: The Synergetic Geometry of R. Buckminster Fuller by Amy Edmonson ed. Arthur Loeb Birkhauser Boston Inc., 1986

(18)   http://nycstructuralintegration.com/tensegrity/

(19)   Tensegrity: Introduction to Theory and Model construction by Robert Grip Buckminster Fuller Institute 1978

(20)   http://www.intensiondesigns.com/geometry_of_anatomy.html

(21)   Frymoyer J W, Pope M H, Wilder D G 1990 Segmental instability. In: Weinstein J N, Wiesel S (eds) The lumbar spine. S aunders, Philadelphia, PA, pp 612-636

(22)   Gardner-Morse M, Stokes I A F, Lauble J P 1995 Role of the muscles in lumbar spine stability in maximum extension efforts. Journal of Orthopaedic Research 13:802-808 Gardner-Morse M G, Stokes I A 1998 The effects of abdominal muscle coactivation on lumbar spine stability. Spine 23:86-91

(23)   "intrinsically." American Heritage® Dictionary of the English Language, Fifth Edition. 2011. Houghton Mifflin Harcourt Publishing Company 22 Mar. 2015 http://www.thefreedictionary.com/intrinsically

SECTION 3

THE
CONTRIBUTING
STATISTICS

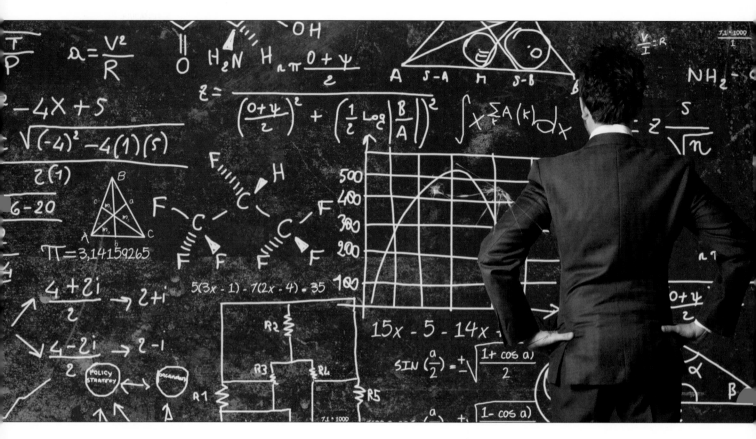

As our modern lifestyle has become more sedentary over the past 75 years, the number of musculo-skeletal disorder cases has risen significantly. Musculo-skeletal disorders are defined as any form of chronic pain in the connective tissues, joints, muscles, and tendons. These disorders are extremely common in the neck, back, feet, ankles, knees and hands and include arthritis, disc herniation, joint degeneration, tendinitis and sciatica. According to the Council of Disability Awareness, the largest cause of new (28.5%) and pre-existing (30.7%) disability claims in 2012 were musculo-skeletal disorders. Shockingly, over 2.5 million of these disabled workers were between the ages of 20 and 40. How can so many young people have these issues with chronic pain?

How did young adults become so receptive to pain?

Too Much Sitting and Not Enough Moving

We can agree that there is a correlation between excessively sedentary lifestyles and an increased rate of musculo-skeletal disorders. People are commonly spending up to 70% of their day sitting. With a sedentary lifestyle and a stationary approach to exercise, the entire body is rarely challenged or trained to work in natural dynamic positions. This lack of movement limits the circulation of blood, nutrients, fluids and oxygen throughout the body, leading to muscular atrophy—the physical loss of muscle mass—in the body's important stabilizing muscles.

As some of the muscles and joints degenerate (break down over time), it becomes increasingly difficult for the body to support itself and equally distribute weight. When human bodies move without symmetrical and synergistic muscle control, it is rare to find proper joint alignment. Improper joint control increases the rate of joint tissue degeneration, directly increasing the risk of developing arthritis, osteoporosis, spondylosis and disc damage/herniation. Poor muscle control will ultimately cause a greater probability of consistent pain.[23, 24, 25, 40]

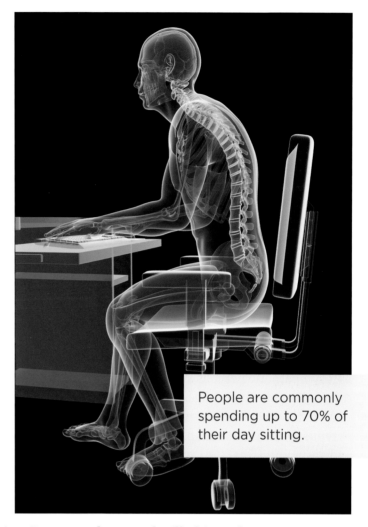

People are commonly spending up to 70% of their day sitting.

Too Much Stress

Constant tension from mental stress also plays an important role. Left unchecked, the pressures of modern life can cause a constant state of mental stress. Constant stress can effect our breathing patterns and directly change the state of the nervous system. Excessive mental stress can cause unnatural and inappropriate breathing patterns. Normally, we should take heavy chest breaths during maximal physical challenges like high intensity workouts, fighting, running, and being scared half to death. These instances require heavy, rapid chest breaths which also stimulate the sympathetic nervous system. The sympathetic nervous system ensures that the body is in a heightened state of awareness, and is designed to make us ready for action. This state is commonly referred to as the "fight or flight" mode, an excellent natural defense mechanism when needed.

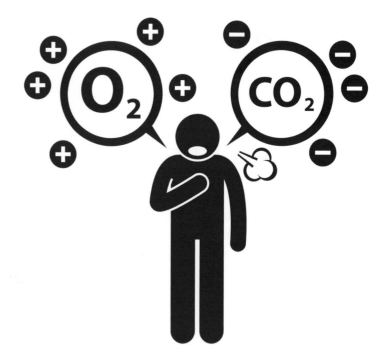

Without proper deep breathing, it can easily take our bodies up to four hours to calm down after entering the "fight or flight" mode. If we even let ourselves calm down, excessive and continuous mental stress will prevent us from entering a parasympathetic state. Health issues arise when the sympathetic nervous system stays continually active throughout the day. Short, rapid chest breathing, elevated blood sugar, elevated heart rate, and excessive alertness are not meant to be experienced all day, everyday, week after week. Staying in this state for a prolonged period can overwhelm and fatigue the body. [26]

Not Enough Quality Rest

The body must have periods of real rest consisting of mental and physical relief. During rest, the parasympathetic nervous system allows the body to repair and regenerate, in a process commonly referred to as "rest and digest". As we breathe from the diaphragm—breathing from the belly instead of from the chest—the parasympathetic nervous system is activated. When the parasympathetic nervous system is dominant, the heart rate is lower, the body conserves energy. The salivary glands and gastrointestinal (GI) tract are stimulated to more efficiently break food down and absorb the micronutrients needed to continuously nourish and repair the body.

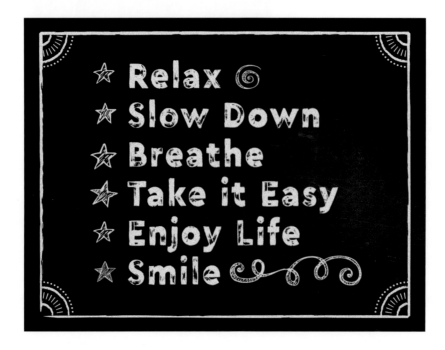

INTRINSIC STRENGTH TRAINING

When the stress of life starts to erode your mental state, sit back and take a few deep breaths. Spending a few minutes deep breathing or meditating throughout the day can significantly improve how you feel. Some musculo-skeletal problems are at least partially caused by a lack of mental and physical rest. Consistent mental stress over prolonged periods of time will begin to create chronic muscular tension through the body, especially the neck, upper back, and hips. When excess muscle tension restricts the range of motion in these areas, the joints are unable to move as designed. The excess tension also restricts circulation, causing joint dehydration. To repair and restore your body, remember to change your nervous system mode to "rest and digest" throughout the day. Leave your "fight and flight" mode for the gym, running away from danger, and closing deals!

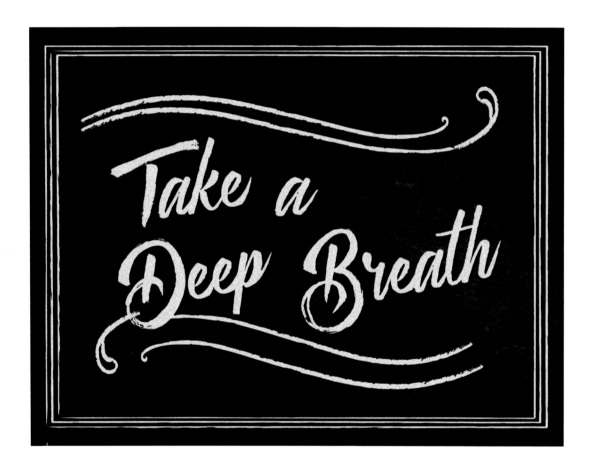

INTRINSIC STRENGTH TRAINING

CHAPTER 9

We Are Only as Strong as Our Weakest Links

Each year, back pain prevents millions of Americans from experiencing the joys of an active lifestyle. The most common cause of back pain is spondylosis—the degeneration (excessive wear and tear) of the spinal vertebrae and the discs between them. Excess stress from poor joint control causes the soft tissue of the spinal segments to lose their natural shape, leading to consistent and reoccurring back pain.

Is there a correlation between chronic back pain and how well you can or can't control your body as one integrated unit? Spending thousands of hours in a stagnant seated position each year is a contributing factor to pain-related issues and reoccurring injuries. Avoiding daily physical activity will result in poor body control. With poor body control comes an increased risk of injury and joint degeneration because the body lacks a full range of motion, core strength, and balance. Distributing imposed forces successfully throughout the entire body with safe joint alignment is nearly impossible with a weak core—even distributing the body's own weight can become a challenge.

Similarly, poor overall body control leads to a weaker and injury prone body. Low back pain—from injury or inactivity—is debilitating and can completely suck the joy from your daily life. Improving your life may only require some daily physical effort. Building a healthy body starts with becoming active.

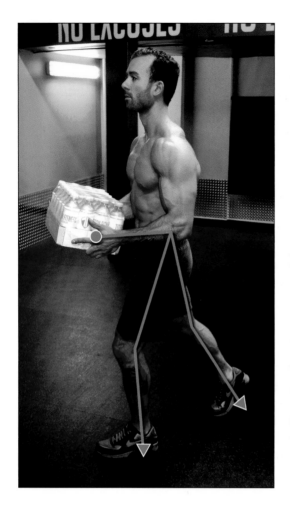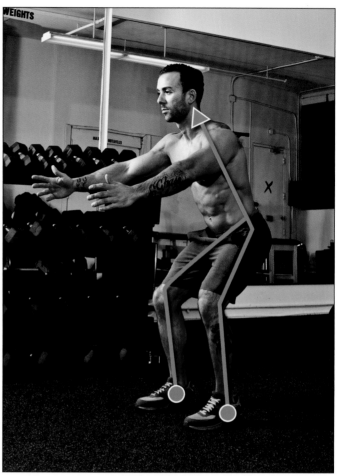

Do you think that extreme joint degeneration and chronic pain after the age of 20 should seem normal for a human body that has evolved for over a six million years? It does not seem right... But, as sedentary lifestyles become more prevalent today—along with increased disability and back pain, it seems like *poor body control and inactivity could be the cause of this epidemic.*

Sitting for extended periods of time has many downsides. First, a chair provides continuous stability for the body, and unlike standing, sitting does not require every muscle to support the entire body. The decreased muscular activity during prolonged periods of extremely passive, rounded seated positions also decreases blood flow throughout the core and extremities. Less muscle activity and decreased blood flow lead to dehydrated and malnourished joints, tendons, muscles, and all forms of connective tissue. Lack of hydration and nourishment can negatively affect the health of every part of your body. Joints, tendons, muscles, nerves, connective tissue all require consistent hydration and nourishment to properly repair themselves.

Using every muscle through a full range of motion increases circulation throughout the entire body. This increased circulation will nourish and hydrate the deeper tissue layers, creating a stronger, healthier body. With restricted ranges of motion, the quality of circulation is limited. Decreased blood flow and dehydration weaken the body.

Is Core Instability a Major Factor of Joint Pain?

More sitting limits the core's muscular activity and blood flow. When the core is not used, it is less nourished, less healthy, unconditioned, and generally less physically able. If the core is unconditioned, it will be more difficult for it to provide the tonic (continuous) tension needed for proper spinal alignment as the body moves. If the muscles of the core are too weak, it may be impossible to maintain healthy spinal alignment.

A weak core is unstable, with less joint stability and inefficient muscle control through the pelvis, segments of the spine, and shoulders. Without core stability, the body will never reach its full physical potential, ultimately leading to poor posture, excessive muscle tension and chronic pain. [11]

Every segment (vertebra) of the spine is required to move during all forms of locomotion. As the muscles of the entire body are integrated, the muscles of the deep core provide a stable base of constant tension for the spine. This stable foundation is only possible with consistent joint control and stability. Without it, the body will always be one small uncontrolled step away from injury. [10, 11, 13, 20, 21]

Efficient full body muscle control is only possible when the segments of the spine move fluidly with the extremities through all upright activity. Many layers of core musculature must work together to provide muscular support for the spine. In a recent study, subjects trained using full body movements and loaded resistance to improve the "corset reaction" of the core. This training directly teaches the muscles of the core to stabilize the pelvis and spine together while efficiently controlling the extremities as they reacted to external resistance. Efficient, unrestricted, and healthy corset reaction (core tension) resulted in the relief of low back pain symptoms and the prevention of recurrent back pain. [28, 29, 30]

Could your Foundation be Your Weak Link?

Within the body's natural tensegrity structure, a local force can affect the entire structure. If there is a local pain or problem, it can affect the function of the entire body.

An unstable—or weak—core can directly limit the performance and safety of the upper and lower extremities by failing to maintain proper joint alignment during all forms of locomotion. A "weak core" fails to provide the constant tension needed to control and stabilize the spine while the body moves. Every force imposed on the body will challenge the core's stability.

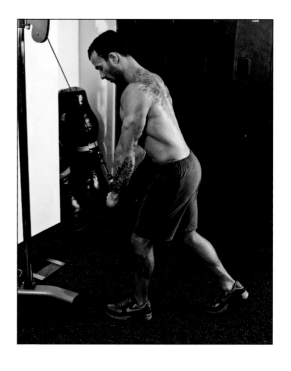

Question: How did my core become weak?

Answer: Extensive periods of sitting, repetitive seated and assisted exercise, lack of dynamic training, lack of daily physical activity, and prior injury.

Listen to Pain

Most people will usually choose to avoid inflicting pain on themselves, but sometimes pain is completely unavoidable. Painful experiences are usually an indirect consequence, and not a directly chosen outcome.

Fear is commonly associated with back pain, and sufferers will hesitate or refuse to try any activities which are physical or new.

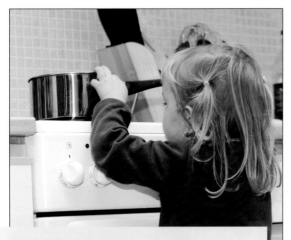

We easily learn or remember to not touch a hot object again.
We choose to avoid something that we know will hurt.

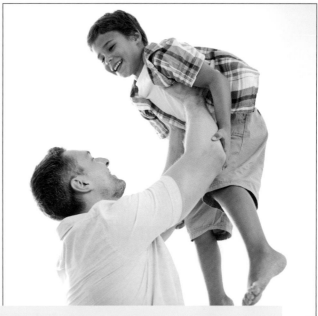

Would you let a weak core keep you from picking up after and playing with your child or pet?

Do not accept this pain, improve your life experiences by strengthening your core and improving your body's functionality. It is no secret that the degeneration of a joint's connective tissue will lead to pain. Are you ignoring the pain that may be indicating a problem with the function of your body or core? Carefully observe pain when it occurs, and consciously evaluate your movements and actions.

Fitness is not only about showing off a well-earned physique, but should also allow you to bring the joy of movement back into your life.

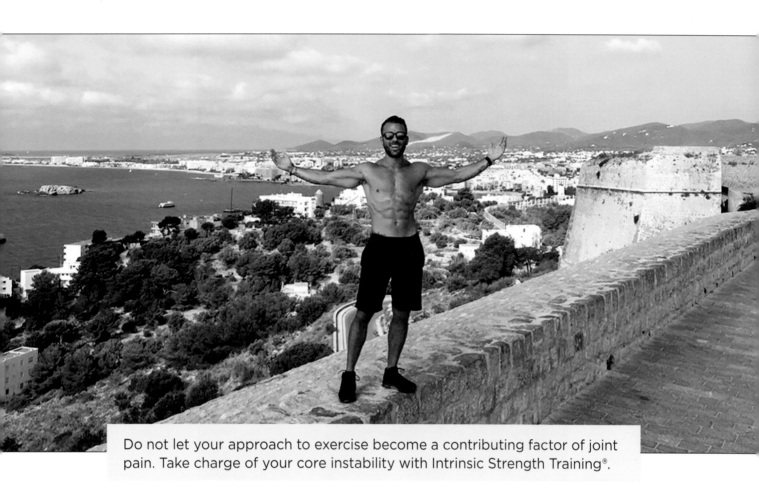

Do not let your approach to exercise become a contributing factor of joint pain. Take charge of your core instability with Intrinsic Strength Training®.

To be clear, sitting is not ideal for the human spine, especially with added resistance. While in a seated position, the lumbar spine (the lowest section of the spine) is fully flexed, which contributes to excessive stress on the discs and can predispose them for herniation.

The best posture is dynamic, and will require more muscle and brain activity .

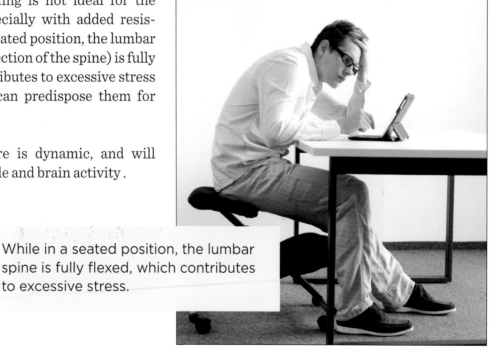

While in a seated position, the lumbar spine is fully flexed, which contributes to excessive stress.

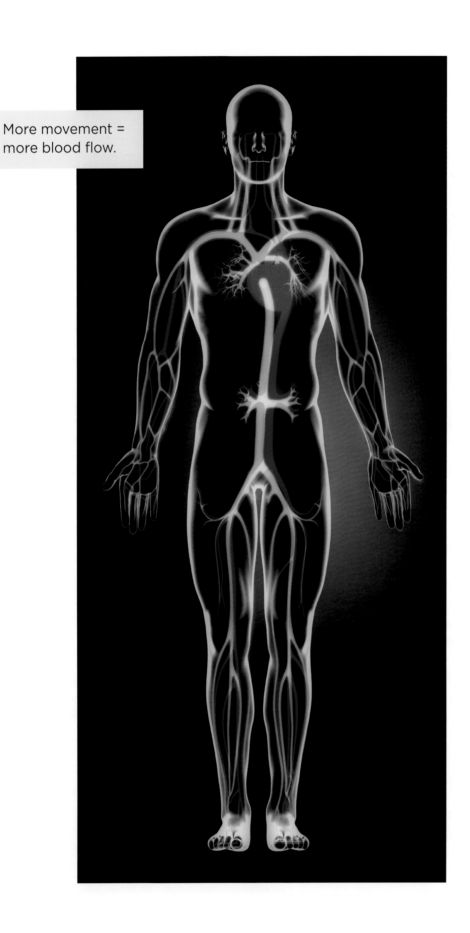

More movement =
more blood flow.

INTRINSIC STRENGTH TRAINING

CHAPTER 10

With Repetition Comes Replication

The SAID principle—Specific Adaptation to Imposed Demands—states that the body will adapt to the specific demands which are repetitively experienced. When the body is challenged by a repetitive stressor, it must adapt to accommodate the physical and mental requirements.

- Muscles grow and become denser after muscle tissue is repetitively broken down from exercise or other activities.
- Bone can also adapt to repetitive stress. For example, bunions form when osteoblast cells are sent to increase bone density in response to repetitive stimulus at the big toe joint. As the first metatarsal (big toe) repetitively strikes the ground, bone-making cells will grow to increase that bone's density.
- Great skills are learned through repetitive stress and practice.

Bones, ligaments, tendons, and muscles can become thicker, denser and stronger when repetitively challenged. However, these same connective tissues can also atrophy from improper training or lack of use.

1. Muscles grow
2. Structures change

Over time, the body can structurally transform to prepare for future challenges, and learn individual tasks and motor patterns.

Simply put, our bodies get better at what we spend time doing.

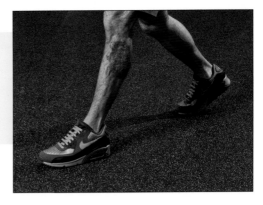

What skills are you interested in improving?
Are you interested in being really great at sitting and standing still, or are you interested in moving better on your feet?

We are dynamic creatures, and Intrinsic Strength Training® uses dynamic exercise to create a joyful workout experience. IST will challenge and improve your movement patterns by improving your ability to control your body.

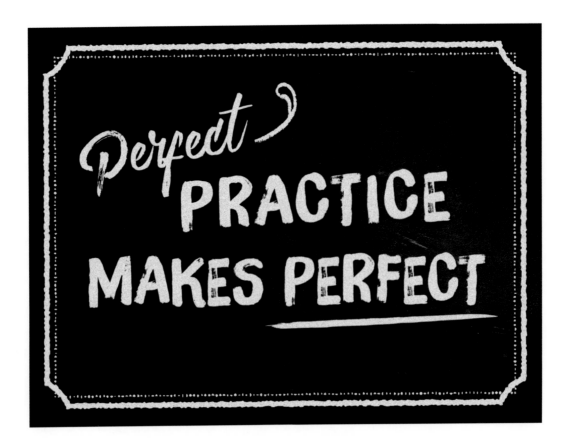

INTRINSIC STRENGTH TRAINING

The Process of Successful Motor Learning

Our bodies and minds are in a constant state of evaluation, reaction and learning. We can remember movement patterns. Have you ever noticed how effortless and instinctual walking seems? Walking is a learned motor pattern. Our bodies also remember positive and negative actions, reactions, and feelings.

For example, consider the process of learning to ride a bicycle. When I first learned to ride without training wheels, I remember jerking the handlebars to the left very quickly. Then the next thing I knew, I was on the ground with the wind knocked out of me! The moral of the story? I never jerked the handlebars to the left like that again! I instantly learned not to repeat that same motor pattern unless I wanted to experience failure and pain.

Do you remember the first time you tried rock climbing? If you lacked integrated full body strength, moving from peg to peg was most likely an unsuccessful experience. Some beginners shake uncontrollably, or become so tense that they can't move at all. But if you are committed to trying a few more times, you will probably start to experience success. With repetition, your mind and body will learn to work efficiently, allowing you to move more freely and finally climb up a few pegs. The process of motor learning can directly improve your rock climbing experience.

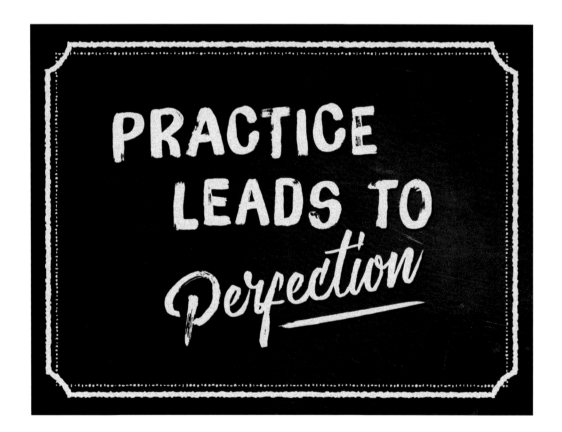

Motor learning improves our capabilities and accuracy through repetitive movement practice.

The natural process of motor learning is designed to work in our favor. Learning how to walk is a monumental challenge for a baby. But as adults, it is effortless and completely automatic since we have spent so much time walking. Each part of the body will remember how to work together for any movements we repeat.

The process of motor learning has three phases. Each phase improves coordination and control, making each individually practiced movement pattern more efficient over time. The three stages of learning are cognitive, associative, and autonomous.

The cognitive first stage requires constant concentration, attention, and focus through the entire task or movement. Multi-tasking will be nearly impossible and performance quality (shakiness, lack of balance, a need to "bail out") will be inconsistent in this phase.

With repetition, we progress to the second stage, the associative phase. Our understanding of the task (movement pattern) and control will improve. As the body becomes more efficient and shakes less, the task will become much easier, and with a higher rate of success. This phase still requires constant attention and will have some spots of inconsistent quality.

With even more repetition and practice we progress to the third stage, the autonomous phase. Now the task becomes habitual and automatic. As the task (movement pattern) is learned, consistent success becomes much easier. After reaching this phase of an exercise or movement pattern, it is time to increase the difficulty or challenge. Repetitive movement patterns can be learned.

Remember, exercise consists of repeating movements. With each exercise, we can improve our movement quality and replicate similar movement patterns outside the gym.

MOTOR LEARNING:

1. The process of acquiring a skill by which the learner, through practice and assimilation, refines and makes the desired movement automatic"? Derek, make this change.
2. An internal neurologic process that results in the ability to produce a new motor task. (34)

We can learn both beneficial and damaging movement patterns inside and outside the gym. Depending on muscle coordination, if our training patterns are inconsistent with the required behavior or activity, a NEGATIVE transfer is likely to occur—for example, continually training the body while in a seated or assisted position. But with practice, we can teach ourselves to do anything. We possess the amazing ability to instantly show signs of improvement at any task.

Where It Counts

A successful and efficient movement pattern will provide each muscle with the perfect amount of tension to keep every joint in perfect alignment as the body moves. In contrast, an inefficient or incorrect movement pattern will cause a disruption in the body's flow.

We can train our bodies to become extremely tense or incredibly passive. The key to movement success is continually finding a balance between these two states. The body can become tense enough to restrict joint movement when an external force is imposed on the body, but excessive tightness can also limit overall body movement. Yet, if we are passive enough that the joints can be controlled and manipulated by external forces, we lose the ability to control and stabilize the alignment of our joints. This results in poor body control, weakness, and a lack of muscular tension.

Set yourself up for success by challenging the body to move in between tension and relaxation.

Since the body learns and adapts to what it does repetitively, have you questioned your approach to exercise and resistance training?

When continually using Intrinsic Strength Training®, the body have the ability to move upright with different points of resistance. IST will improve your movement competency within an upright dynamic environment. IST teaches real world strength and mobility. You will feel a dramatic improvement in your balance and coordination.

During the first few weeks of IST, you will certainly feel an improvement in stability and balance as your core strengthens and integrates with the rest of your body.

Are you only interested in feeling balanced or coordinated while seated or lying down? Are you interested in using fewer muscles while limiting your physical abilities and burning fewer calories?

Of course not!

INTRINSIC STRENGTH TRAINING

CHAPTER 11

Involving More of the Core with Intrinsic Strength Training®

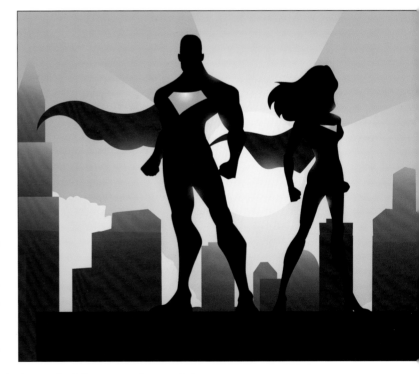

Body language is the largest factor of human communication. During a conversation, 55% of what we perceive is body language. Posture can communicate wellbeing, social hierarchy, stress, and confidence.[36] Does someone with a slouched posture and awkward body language appeal to you? A slouching, stiff, poor posture is usually associated with disinterest or a lack of confidence.[35]

Suffering from poor body control can limit your life in bigger ways outside of sports. I learned about the NARP (Non-Athletic Regular People) label from a few Division 1 sports athletes. It's how they describe people with poor posture and who walk with poor movement quality. A typical NARP has poor posture, poor joint control, excessive muscle stiffness, joint pain, limited physical abilities, and complaints.

Which posture is most approachable ?

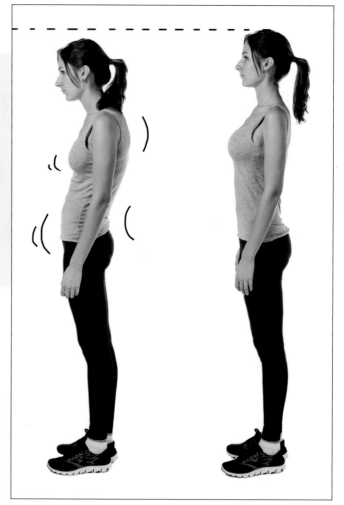

Are you interested in a life of poor posture, poor interactions, and possibly being misinterpreted during conversation? Or would you rather have a confident posture, more meaningful interactions, and memorable experiences? Having excellent control of your body feels good and brings joy back into your day.

A strong and stable core is essential for a confident posture and an able body. When the body's fluid integration is disrupted by core weakness and joint instability, the efficiency and quality of body control is directly effected.

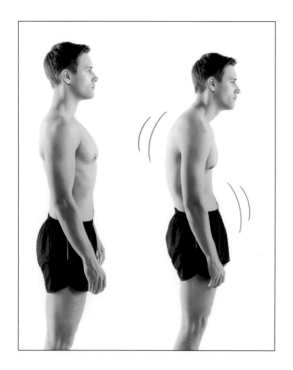

Have you ever seen a bodybuilder or fitness model who looks super fit and muscular? You might automatically assume that they are very strong or fit—but sadly most of them have accomplished their impressive visual results while sitting down. These impressive physical specimens may look strong, but most of their strength is limited to a few select exercises in the gym. These exercises are usually performed while remaining in one static position or with the assistance of a bench or machine. So, most of these aesthetically trained people suffer from poor body control, balance problems, a weak functional core, and lower back pain.

I've personally met countless people who look strong and have a ripped 6 pack—but who also have an extremely weak core. In fact, years ago, I was one of them.

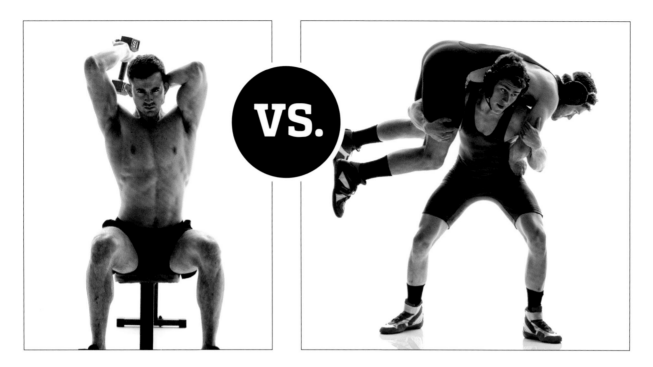

I've transformed myself from "all show and no go" to someone with excellent body control and useable full body strength. Through this experience, I came up with three big questions:

- Think about the last time you were challenged with a strenuous movement-based task. Did you actually feel confident in your ability to complete it?
- Have you spent countless hours in the gym limiting your physical strength to seated, lying, or stationary positions?
- When faced with a strenuous physical challenge outside the gym, did you use a chair to help you complete the task?

We can fix these problems with our approach:

- Stop training the body to work without including the entire body in the exercise!
- Stop relying on a chair or bench to help stabilize your body during exercise—the core should engage and provide a stable foundation!
- Add stepping patterns to your resistance training to replicate how we continually step to move.

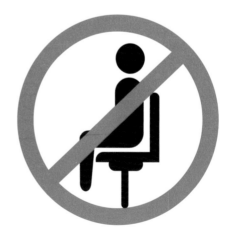

Multi-positional strength is a necessity. We will always need to physically move throughout the day. If each workout challenges your ability to dynamically control your body, your abilities to move your body throughout the day will improve.

Along with achieving aesthetic goals, a workout should improve your ability to control and balance your own body.

Intrinsic Strength Training® demands the greatest involvement of the multiple muscular layers of the core with every upright, unilateral exercise. For example, when doing a unilateral overhead press, there is 81% more activity in the rectus abdominis as compared to a bilateral overhead press. When standing, 59% more muscular activity occurs compared to sitting. [36, 37, 38, 39]

Intrinsic Strength Training® requires changing positions during each exercise. The muscles throughout the whole body and core are required to integrate with the extremities.
The quality of this integration directly affects how well the body can generate the perfect amount of tension to stabilize and move.

Upright and unilateral training also requires more activity within the primary muscle group for a given exercise. When performing an upright unilateral dumbbell shoulder press, the anterior, lateral, and posterior deltoid all required more muscular activation while standing as opposed to performing a seated shoulder press with a barbell, using both arms (36,37,38,39)

Front shoulder (anterior deltoid) EMG results for seated dumbbell vs. standing dumbbell press: muscle activation was 8% greater for the standing dumbbell press.

Middle shoulder (lateral deltoid) EMG results for seated dumbbell vs. standing barbell press: muscle activation was 7% greater for the standing barbell press.

Back shoulder (posterior deltoid) EMG results for seated dumbbell vs. standing dumbbell press: muscle activation was 24% greater for the standing dumbbell press.)

CHAPTER 12

The 10 Commandments of Intrinsic Strength Training

Do you want to maximize your results during a workout, create a symmetrical physique, improve your balance, strength, and full body control? Then promise yourself that you will no longer limit your full potential by exercising in a seated or lying position. No more sitting on a machine, lying on a bench, or peddling while hunched over a cardio bike.

An ideal training program consists of a complete repertoire of full body movements that stress multi-directional control.

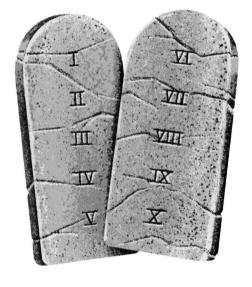

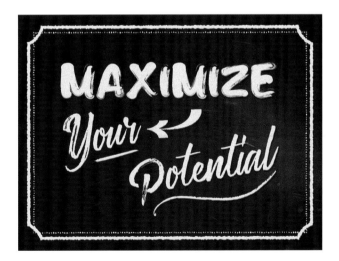

The body is more advanced than a precision-tuned performance car, and when used to its full potential, the brain is more powerful than any supercomputer. Let's start using our bodies the way they were designed to perform.

Anyone wanting to build Intrinsic Strength® will need to follow these 10 commandments:

1st Commandment:
You Shall Acknowledge the Whole is Greater than the Sum of Its Parts (Aristotle)

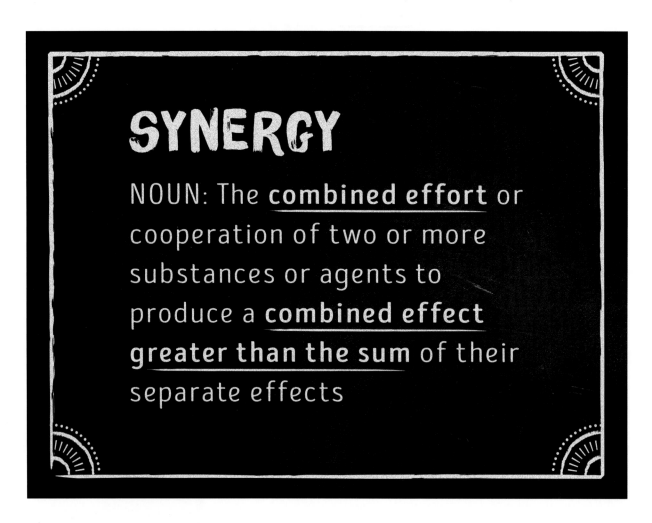

SYNERGY

NOUN: The **combined effort** or cooperation of two or more substances or agents to produce a **combined effect greater than the sum** of their separate effects

While standing upright, we can observe the following:

- As we step forward with each leg, each step will change the orientation of the hips.
- As we reach to the side with either arm, reaching will change the position of our shoulders.

We know the pelvis and spine are connected. We know that the arms influence the shoulders. We know that the legs influence the pelvis . If the pelvis, spine, and shoulders are interconnected layers of connective tissue, then whenever the arms or legs move, the position of the shoulder and pelvis change. When the pelvis or shoulders move, the vertebrae of the spine move with them. When the bones are moving, then the muscles are active and moving!

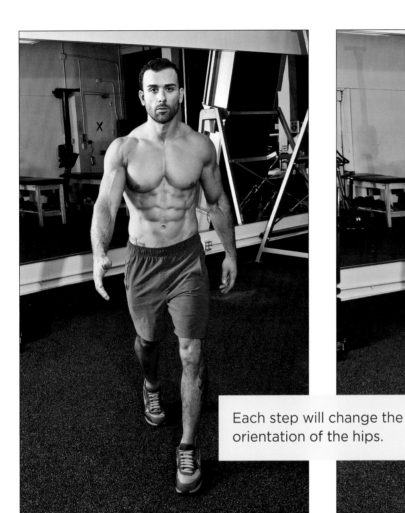

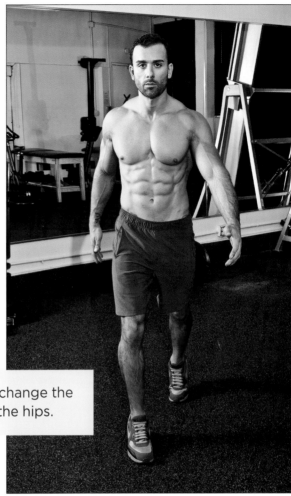

Each step will change the orientation of the hips.

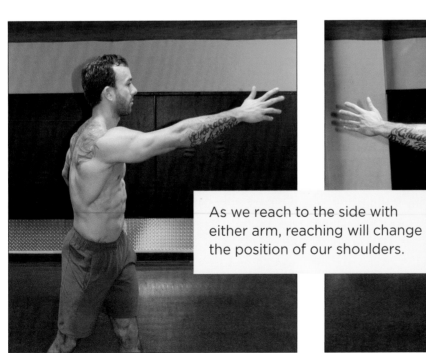

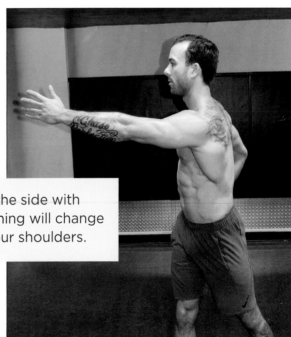

As we reach to the side with either arm, reaching will change the position of our shoulders.

The extremities and core are unified in one integrated structure. About 630 muscles and 206 bones are required to operate the 230 joints of the human body with precise control. When your body possesses the muscular strength to adequately control all ranges of motion then you can develop great physical abilities.

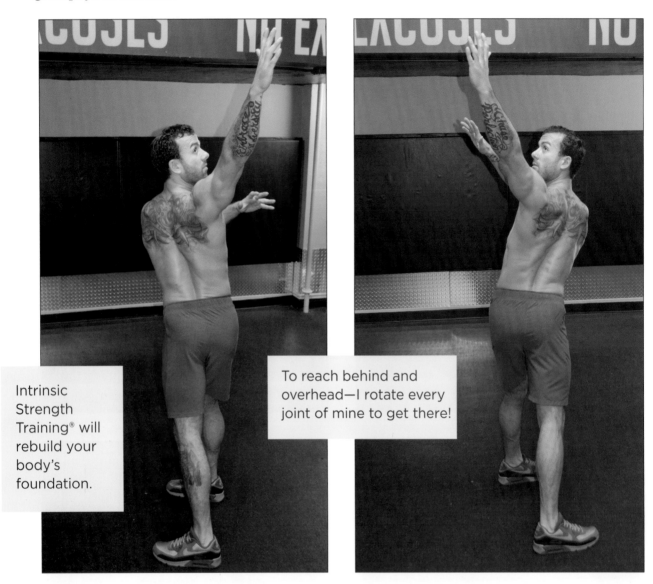

Intrinsic Strength Training® will rebuild your body's foundation.

To reach behind and overhead—I rotate every joint of mine to get there!

Precise body control is only possible with a stable foundation—the core. The deepest layers of the core provide constant tension to the spine, providing a stable base to radiate muscular tension outward into the extremities. The quality of your foundation relies on your lifestyle, nutrition, and approach to exercise.

2nd Commandment:
You Shall Not Associate Sitting with Fitness, but with Weakness

Fitness is much more complex than simply determining how many reps you can do, how much weight you can lift, and how fast you can do it while in a seated or stationary position. Fitness goes deeper than a bathroom ab selfie. Important factors of an active lifestyle are improving your body's longevity and abilities, which leads to an exciting and enjoyable physical life.

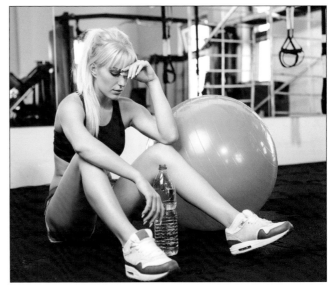

So, why not maximize your physical potential? Most fun activities—and even chores—are rarely done sitting down or standing still, yet our approach to exercise is often sitting down and standing still. If we know extensive periods of sitting is bad for us, then why are we spending so much time doing it? Every day we are required to move without the assistance of a chair, so why are we associating fitness and exercise with chairs, seats, benches, or machines?

Do you need to rely on the assistance of a chair or machine to exercise? Are your legs and core too weak to support the weights that you can hold in your hands?

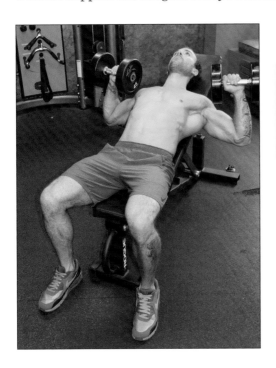

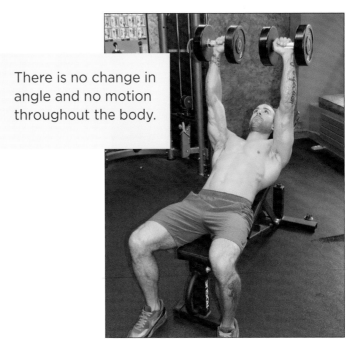

There is no change in angle and no motion throughout the body.

We are humans—the most biologically advanced species on this planet—let's start exercising like it.

Intrinsic Strength Training® will continually challenge the body with upright multi-dimensional dynamic unilateral exercise. With IST, the body works as one unit, improving balance, coordination, muscle symmetry, dynamic strength, joint control, and health.

3rd Commandment:
You Shall Continually Challenge Your Base of Support (BOS)

Within our daily lives, we must get from "point A" to "point B" by taking continuous steps. Throughout the day, the average person takes about 4,000 to 12,000 steps. Each step requires the integrated effort of the entire body as the upper and lower extremities move simultaneously.

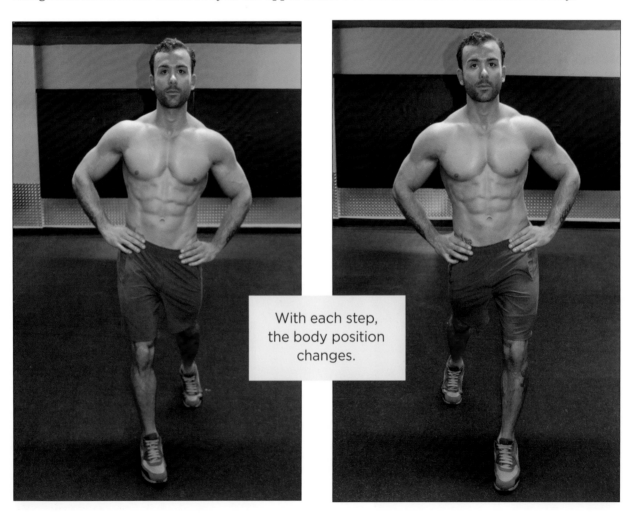

With each step, the body position changes.

Unfortunately, conventional approaches to exercise fail to replicate how we move in real life. Resistance training usually disregards the simultaneous upper and lower extremity control we need when we move. Only rarely do we have to take large steps into deep lunges or perfectly aligned squats during our normal daily activities. Our usual steps are small, multi-directional, and continuous.

For example, think about cooking a family meal in the kitchen. This task requires going back and forth to the refrigerator, the sink and the food preparation area in no particular order. Getting to each area of the kitchen will require different types of steps. There is also a simultaneous integration of the upper and lower extremities while bending and reaching into the oven, rotating and reaching up into the cabinets, and reaching deep into back of the fridge. Our approach to fitness should replicate and challenge our transitions between these different positions.

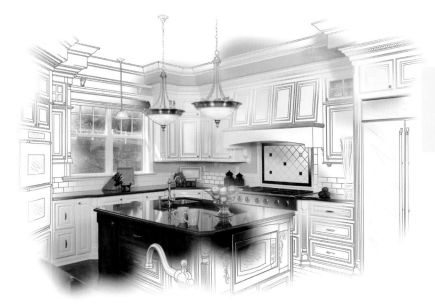

The "work triangle" requires various stepping positions.

When standing upright, our feet are our body's first supports on the ground. The position of our feet will be known as our base of support (BOS). As the BOS changes, the entire body's position will change and challenge different muscles in different ways.

To build the Intrinsic Strength Training® foundation, we need to practice seven basic positions.

1. STARTING (SET UP) POSITION

Our set up position in IST Level 1 is a bilateral stance.

Within Level 1 of Intrinsic Strength Training®, the starting position will always be a bilateral stance, with the feet evenly spaced about shoulder width apart.

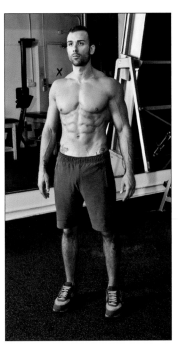

Stand tall, with an actively engaged core and strong posture. When standing upright with any type of resistance, you should feel core engagement. Focus on the integration and alignment of your entire body. Eliminate any excessive pelvic tilting or slouching, so you are prepared to stop excessive forces from leaking directly into the lower back and spine.

Please note that the base of support (BOS) will refer to the foot position and direction of each step during the exercises.

2. FORWARD STEP

Stepping in front of the body, replicating the acceleration stage of walking.

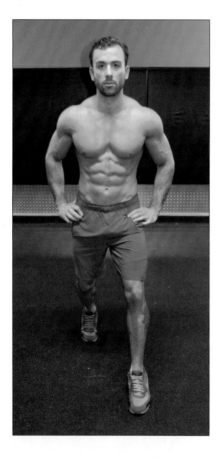 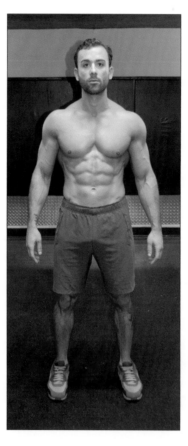 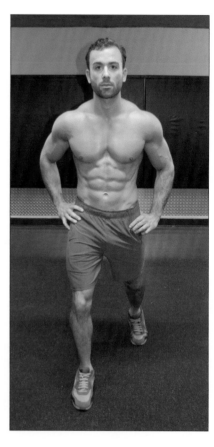

3. REAR STEP

Stepping behind the body

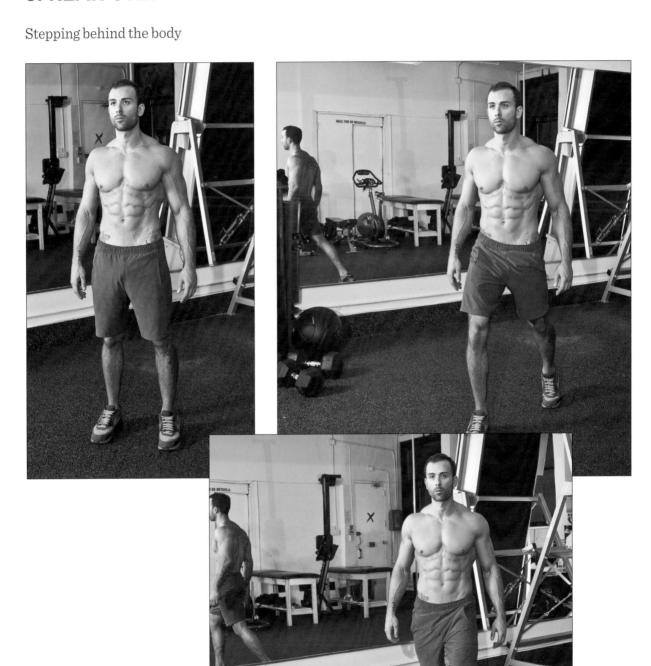

4. LATERAL STEP, LEFT/RIGHT

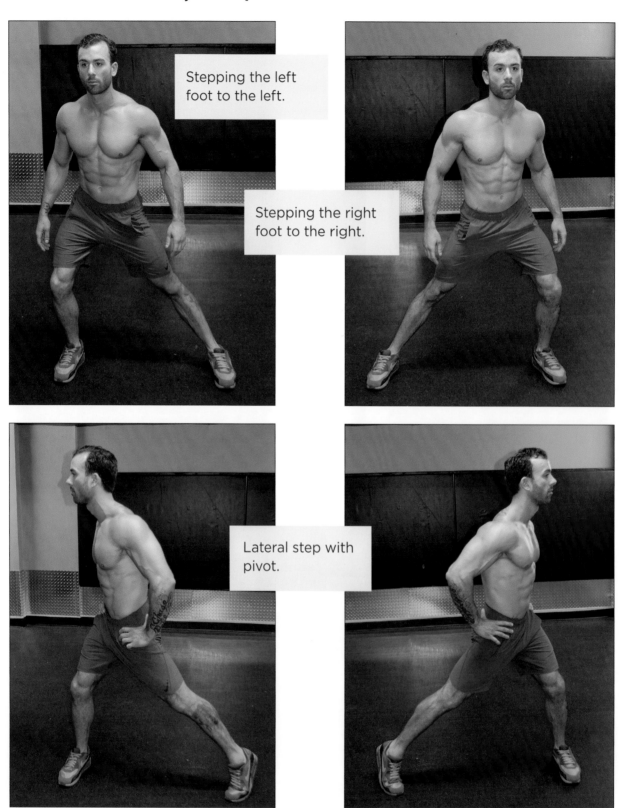

Stepping the left foot to the left.

Stepping the right foot to the right.

Lateral step with pivot.

5. REAR ROTATION STEP

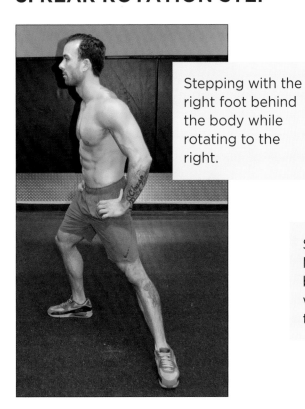

Stepping with the right foot behind the body while rotating to the right.

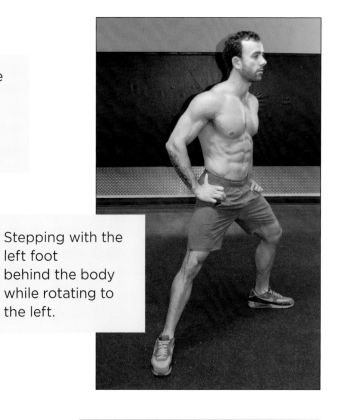

Stepping with the left foot behind the body while rotating to the left.

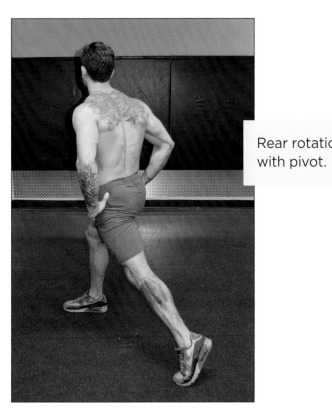

Rear rotation step with pivot.

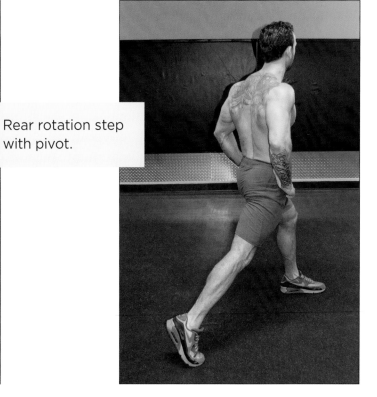

6. CROSSOVER STEP, LEFT/RIGHT

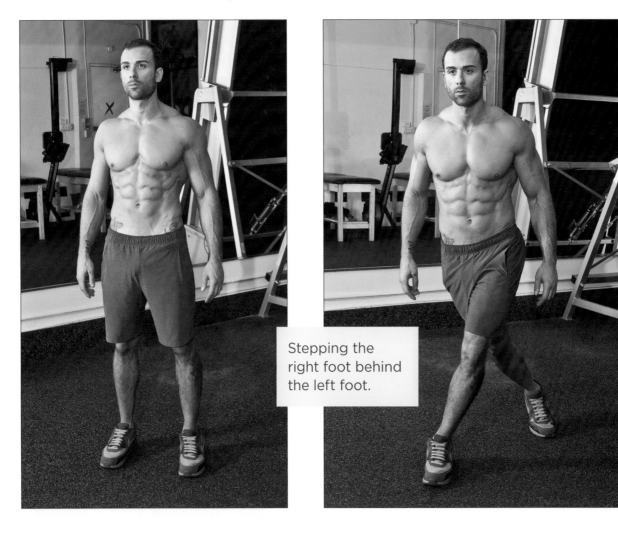

Stepping the right foot behind the left foot.

INTRINSIC STRENGTH TRAINING

4th Commandment:
You Shall Continually Change Your Resistance Location (POR)

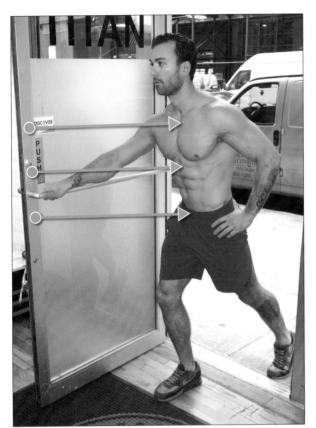

Our lives revolve around our bodies—indisputably, all around our bodies. The physical demands and external forces of life can come from all angles and all positions.

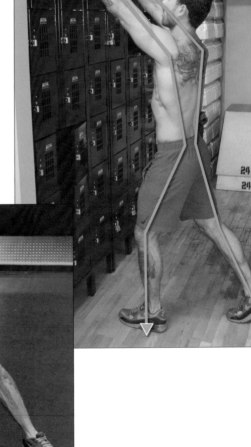

The various resistance locations of IST will continually challenge the body inside the gym to prepare the body for situations outside of the gym. Intrinsic Strength Training® Level 1 challenges the body with one Position of Resistance (POR) for each exercise. POR refers to the changing resistance type, location, and extremity action of each exercise. The POR will indicate how to orient yourself to the resistance point of the exercise, whether the challenge is directly in front, from behind, or from the side.

IST's five resistance heights challenge the body from the ankle, knee, hip, shoulder, and from overhead. The resistance tool used and the extremity action will also be described in POR. IST external resistance items include resistance cables, dumbbells, kettlebells, barbells, as well as body weight only.

1. **Varying Resistance Orientation, Starting Resistance Locations**
   a. Forward Facing
   b. Back Facing
   c. Side Facing

2. **Varying Resistance Heights for Different Reactions**
   a. Ankle
   b. Knee
   c. Hip
   d. Shoulder
   e. Overhead

3. **Resistance Type**
   a. Cable or Band Resistance
      i. One Arm (unilateral)
      ii. Two Arms (bilateral)
   b. Dumbbell or kettlebell
      i. One Arm (unilateral)
      ii. Two Arms (bilateral)
   c. Barbell
      i. Two Arms (bilateral)

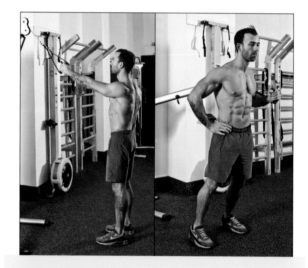

Example of varying resistance orientation, starting resistance locations: forward and backward facing.

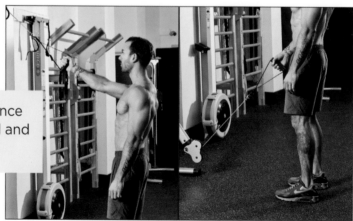

Example of varying resistance heights: showing overhead and ankle height.

5th Commandment:
You Shall Move Your Feet and Hands Simultaneously

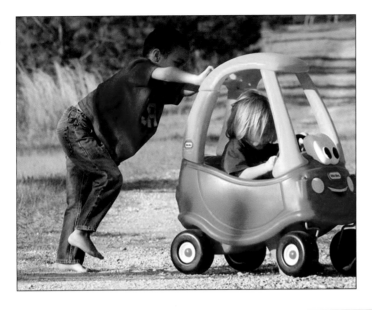

Our most common and universal activity—walking—requires the upper and lower extremities to move simultaneously. Since every upright activity and every form of human locomotion requires the upper and lower extremities to work synergistically, shouldn't our approach to exercise?

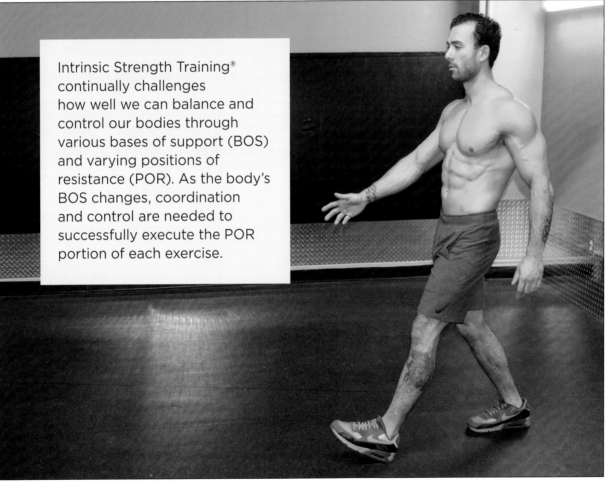

Intrinsic Strength Training® continually challenges how well we can balance and control our bodies through various bases of support (BOS) and varying positions of resistance (POR). As the body's BOS changes, coordination and control are needed to successfully execute the POR portion of each exercise.

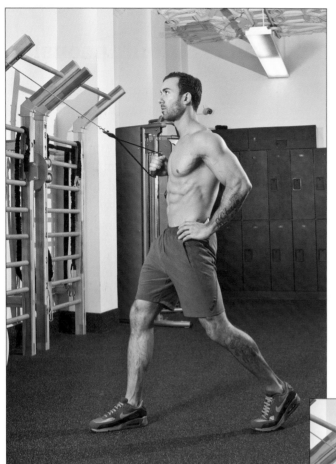

Intrinsic Strength Training® brings dynamic full body motion to classic resistance training exercises. For example, an alternating rear step (BOS) adds motion to a unilateral cable row (POR).

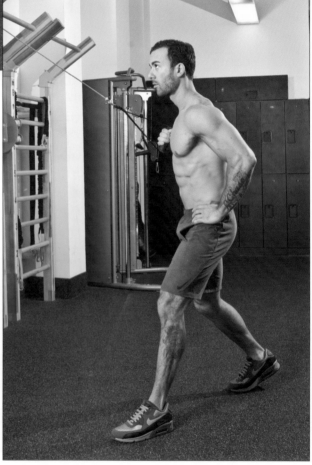

6th Commandment:
You Shall Perform the Three Phases of Each IST Rep

Every Intrinsic Strength Training® exercise rep consists of three phases: dynamic acceleration, global repetition, and dynamic deceleration. Each phase challenges the entire body in a unique way.

1st Phase: Dynamic Acceleration = Dynamic BOS + Concentric POR

The first phase combines a concentric contraction with a step away from the starting position to accelerate the resistance. An example is executing a chest press away from the body while stepping forward. As the body's base of support (BOS) changes with each step, the isolated extremity (POR) will be simultaneously challenged during the concentric phase of the exercise.

The dynamic acceleration phase of IST initiates force production while the body changes position, further requiring the upper and lower extremities to synergistically integrate.

Varying BOS and POR will continually challenge the body to work as a whole, which is essential for many physical activities. Throughout the day, we are often tested when pushing, pulling, lifting, or reaching for something while simultaneously taking a step. We might be pushing open a heavy door, pulling a door shut, pushing a shopping cart, pushing an attacker then running away, picking something up off the floor in mid stride, or reaching for something on the top shelf.

During the day as well as when practicing IST, be mindful of your body's position and control. You will feel when your core is unable to support the resistance while changing the position of your feet.

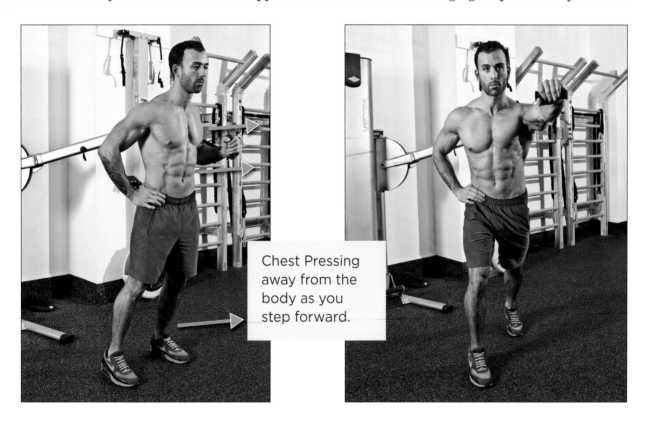

Chest Pressing away from the body as you step forward.

2nd Phase: Global Repetition = Static BOS + Eccentric and Concentric POR

The second phase of the chest press and forward step during the eccentric and concentric phase of the rep is an example of global repetition. It is performed with slight movement throughout the entire body as the feet stay in the same position.

Within this phase, the position of the feet (BOS) is stationary rather than dynamic. During this phase you must control the eccentric and concentric contraction of the localized extremity (POR).

The term "stationary" does not refer to standing perfectly still. In IST, the same rules apply to maintaining your BOS (foot position or stance). The hips and legs are challenged to move against resistance without changing the position of the feet.

You will certainly feel the entire core engage when you focus on applying pressure into the ground through the foot and big toe.

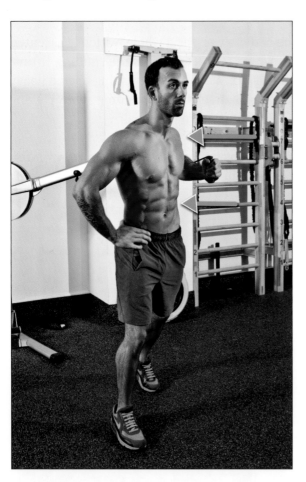 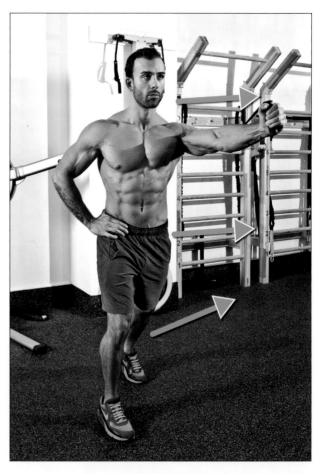

The global repetition phase mimics how our feet sometimes stay in one position as we complete a task with our upper extremities. Examples outside the gym include pulling out a chair to sit down, taking the laundry from the washer and putting it into the dryer, digging and shoveling, unloading the dishwasher, standing your ground while being pushed, and starting a lawn mower or chainsaw.

3rd Phase: Dynamic Deceleration = Dynamic BOS + Eccentric POR

The third phase combines an eccentric contraction, and a step back to the starting position while decelerating the resistance. In our example, this phase's actions would be pulling the chest press back to the body while stepping back to the bilateral starting position. Your feet return to the starting position (BOS) while simultaneously controlling the isolated extremity (POR) through the eccentric phase of the exercise.

The dynamic deceleration phase of IST focuses on returning to the starting position while simultaneously slowing down the momentum of the body and the weight of any external resistance. This phase continues to integrate the upper and lower extremities with the entire body.

When training to decelerate the momentum of the body and added resistance, you are also building up more resistance to injury. We must decelerate every movement we make in life. When bringing something to your chest after pulling it off from an overhead shelf, you wouldn't just let it hit you, you would slow the object down. When running, we don't stop ourselves by running into a wall or other obstacle, we decelerate our momentum with our muscles! When placing a child on the ground, we don't just drop him or her from four feet in the air, we slowly lower them to the ground. (Not like dropping a barbell on the ground after a max deadlift!)

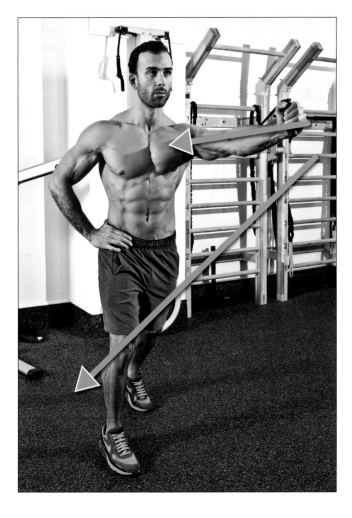
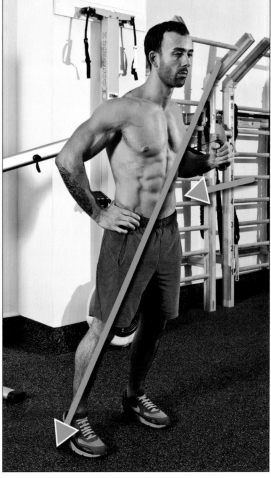

7th Commandment:
You Shall Honor the Three C's of IST

Physical activity will always require precise motor control and coordination. Our approach to exercise must challenge our ability to control and coordinate our bodies.

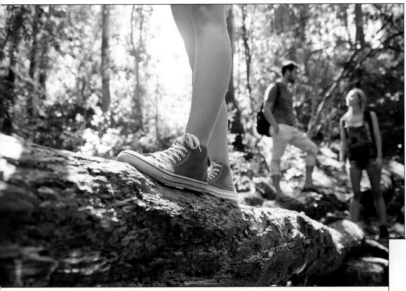

CONTROL

Focus on how well you can control your body. Each IST exercise requires the body to remain stable and balanced through dynamic postures and dynamic and static foot positions. Symmetrical muscle control is essential to a symmetrical physique. All forms of locomotion require continuous joint stability, which is only possible through continuous muscle control.

COORDINATION

Take the time to develop the coordination of each extremity and within the entire body. At first, some exercises will feel significantly more challenging than others. It takes time to learn how to move efficiently in different positions while simultaneously moving your other extremities. These abilities improve over time through the three phases of learning.

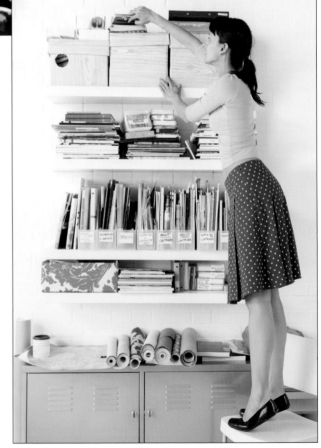

NEVER COMPENSATE

If the resistance is too heavy, and your body moves into an unstable position, you might notice that the movement doesn't "feel right". In that situation, safely return to the starting position. After a short rest, choose a lighter weight and try again. Reps performed under exhaustion usually have poor form which trains poor motor patterns, and can lead to injury. As soon as the body loses the ability to maintain safe joint alignment, please stop the exercise and rest for at least three minutes.

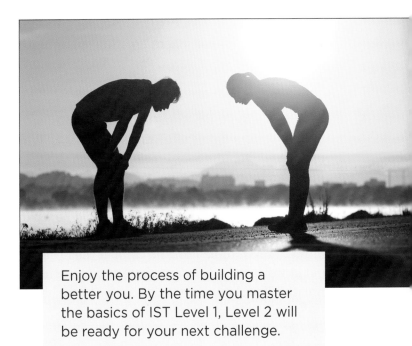

Enjoy the process of building a better you. By the time you master the basics of IST Level 1, Level 2 will be ready for your next challenge.

8th Commandment:
You Shall Breathe for Constant Tension

Creating and maintaining continuous muscular tension while performing multiple IST reps is only possible through continuous breathing. In conventional resistance training, the inhale and exhale are typically timed. Usually, an exhale accompanies the acceleration of the resistance (the concentric contraction of the exercise), then the breath is inhaled with the deceleration of the resistance (the eccentric contraction of the exercise).

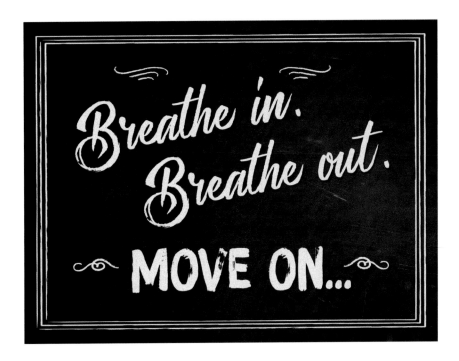

Breathe in.
Breathe out.
~ MOVE ON... ~

In IST, breathing is more than just the inhalation of oxygen and exhalation of carbon dioxide. We want to achieve a consistent breathing pattern which will support constant tension throughout the body. Powerful breathing from the diaphragm will radiate tension through the core to the extremities, providing a stable foundation for all functions.

Integrating our breathing and muscular tension is essential to creating the efficient core tension needed to complete each Intrinsic Strength Training® exercise. Maintaining a regular breathing pattern with continuous tension through the core is also essential for everyday physical activities inside and outside the gym.

Deep, diaphragmatic breathing should be a part of your everyday life. It initiates the repair and rebuilding processes of the parasympathetic nervous system. These processes allow your body and mind to relax, re-center, and combat the negative effects of stress. The next time you are stressed out at work, or become aggravated by someone's actions, try to focus on taking a few big deep belly breaths. You should instantly notice a lower heart rate and less tension throughout your chest.

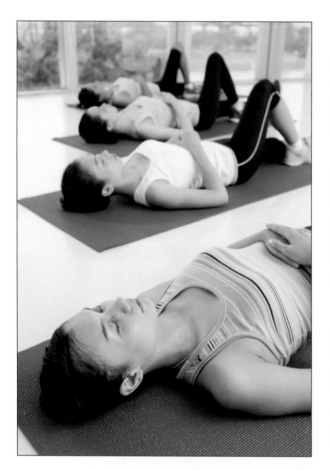

Tensing the core during an activity initiates a strong muscular contraction from the deepest layers of the midsection which radiate through the entire body. When a short burst of maximum strength is needed for a task, bracing will help you produce more strength.

When challenged by a strenuous challenge, I often need to release a little air from my diaphragm to begin bracing. This causes my mouth to make a short hiss or "PSST" sound. Notice how the abdominals and glutes simultaneously tense to provide an extremely stable foundation for maximum strength.

Learning these breathing techniques may be challenging at first. Applying core tension while continuing to breathe can often leave you short of breath. If you find yourself unable to maintain a consistent breathing pattern, lower the weight and focus on your breathing. It's important to avoid shortness of breath which can lead to fainting.

Bracing through the core is used in heavy resistance training such as powerlifting and other explosive and static movements. Under heavy resistance, a challenging rep may require you to contract (squeeze) the abdominals and glutes simultaneously as hard as you can. At the same time, think about squeezing a little bit of air from your belly through your mouth. Bracing with this breathing pattern will create more core tension, and help stabilize the spine during a maximum effort.

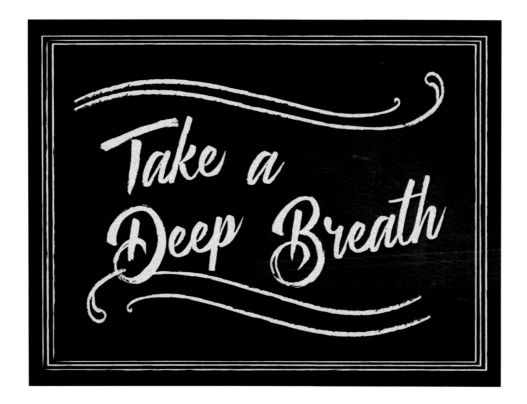

Remember, consciously and continually breathe under control. Do not forget to breathe between moments of bracing.

Try this now:

Inhale deeply through your nose or mouth and allow your entire lower belly to fill up with air before your chest. Next, release all of that air through your mouth. Repeat this breathing pattern for three to five minutes. Now, how do you feel? You may notice that you feel rested, calm, focused, and your heart rate and blood pressure may also be lower.

As you incorporate deep breathing into your daily lifestyle, your stress levels will subside, you will release excess muscular tension, and your body will more easily restore and repair itself.

Before each workout or exercise, take a few very deep breaths. These breaths should fill your entire belly with air before you finally release all of it through your mouth. Belly breathing triggers the body to know it is safe to relax. Initiating the breath from the diaphragm is essential to our physical restoration and focusing processes.

9th Commandment:
You Shall Create Greater Body Control Through Your Big Toe

A machine required to travel on the ground must connect with the ground to move successfully. Different machines connect to varying surface types in many different ways: Tractors have thick knobby tires for traction in sandy or muddy fields. A race car has smooth tread, or "slick" tires for the most possible contact with a flat surface like asphalt. A snowmobile has tracks to move through thick snow.

How well these different machines operate on various types of terrain is entirely dependent on how well they contact each surface. A high powered race car with slick tires would be utterly useless in the snow because the tires do not have treads to gain traction in the snow. Similarly, a snowmobile cannot drive on asphalt.

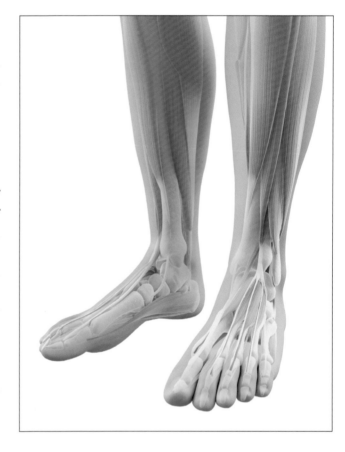

Just like any vehicle, the performance of our human bodies is limited to the quality of our contact with the ground. Since our feet are the first parts of the body to strike the ground, how well they can move will affect how well we can control our whole bodies. Your feet must absorb the force from your body, while also producing the forces to stabilize, and move under control.

Our feet are extremely intricate. Each foot includes twenty-six bones and over 100 muscles, tendons, and nerves.[54] The muscles, tendons, and fascia connecting the big toe, forefoot, and heel continue up the legs and into the core. This structure of connective tissue travels from the big toe and forefoot, wraps around the heel bone, continues up the back side of the leg, though the core and eventually connecting to the skull. This line of connective tissue is referred to as the superficial back line. [41]

Successful walking requires enough mobility in the big toe and foot for free movement while simultaneously providing the appropriate amount of muscle tension for each step. If the big toe and forefoot are too stiff, restricted, or weak (these last two usually occur together) absorbing and propelling the body's weight with proper joint alignment will be extremely difficult.

The same is true for running. It is essential to use the big toe and forefoot with each stride. Absorbing the body's weight with the forefoot is much safer and efficient than striking the ground with the heel. As the forefoot is first to come in contact with the ground, all of the connective tissue of the foot, leg, and core will help distribute the impact of each step—this impact is usually two to four times the runner's body weight. Running by heel striking bypasses the absorption capabilities of the forefoot and leg muscles. With each heel strike, the forces of each stride travel directly

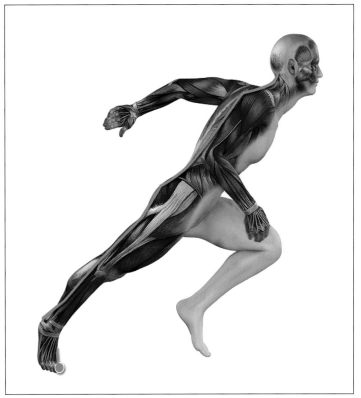

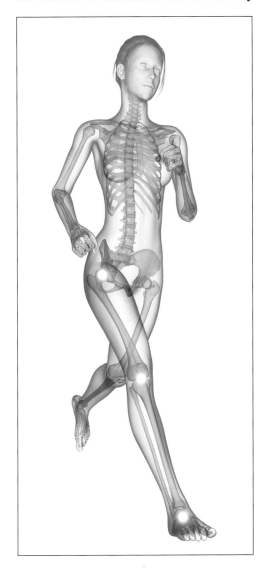

up through the bones and joints instead of distributing the impact through the muscles, tendons, and fascia. Heel striking directs these forces through the heels and into the shins, knees, pelvis and spine.

Runners who continually heel strike will suffer from painful joint inflammation and excess wear and tear from the repetitive high force impacts to the bones and joints. Heel striking can quickly cause acute pain which can progress into chronic pain or a debilitating injury. Instead, distributing the weight and force of each stride through the muscles, tendons, and fascia traveling throughout the foot, legs, and core will limit unnecessary joint and bone stress. Heel striking excessively stresses the joints and bones, including the ankle, tibia (shin), knee, hip, and spine.

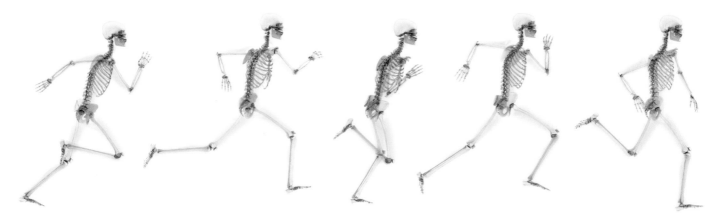

Why Do We Heel Strike?

When the feet and musculature of the lower legs are too weak to absorb the impact of running, heel striking can occur. Heel striking requires less muscular exertion than using the forefoot. Heel striking requires 53% less caloric energy per stride compared to first landing on the forefoot.[29]

Intrinsic Strength Training® exercises are designed to challenge your control over your entire body while activating the core, big toe, and forefoot. To radiate tension throughout the body during all Intrinsic Strength Training® exercises, focus on applying pressure into the ground through the big toe. This focus will enhance how well you can balance, control, and produce the full body power needed for each rep.

10th Commandment:
You Shall Listen to Your Body

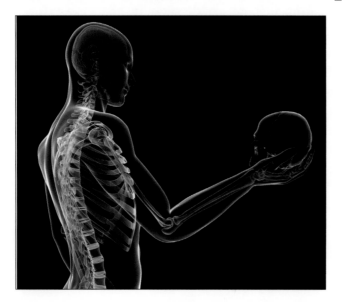

Intuition, gut feelings, joint pains, tender tendons, excessive muscle tension, reoccurring headaches, and fatigue should not be ignored. Our brains and bodies are in a constant state of evaluation and communication. These "random" feelings aren't random. If we don't ignore feelings of hunger or thirst, why do we often ignore these other internal feelings?

The brain is always communicating the present state or status of the body. Millions of proprioceptors throughout the body relay messages to our brain—if we choose to listen to them—while simultaneously controlling the tension and activity of our muscles. The body can quickly evaluate and express feelings of pain, fatigue, sickness, hunger, stress, inflammation, successful integration, overexertion, and injury. Some refer to this as *medical intuition,* which is an awareness of our own physical condition.

If you want to help yourself, start listening to your intuition. Listening to your body can guide you towards taking better care of yourself while understanding what your body needs. Can you relate to any of the following examples of intuition?

EXAMPLE 1:
FEELING THE PHYSICAL EFFECTS OF MENTAL STRESS

After a crazy day at the office, you might leave work feeling extremely stressed, fatigued or overwhelmed. *Your mind might be overly stressed and you may be physically exhausted, but your intuition will always provide multiple warning signals. Did you pick up on them?* You might have had a higher resting heart rate while breathing with shorter, more rapid chest breaths. Instead of deep belly breathing through your diaphragm in a relaxed state, you were preparing your body for "fight or flight".

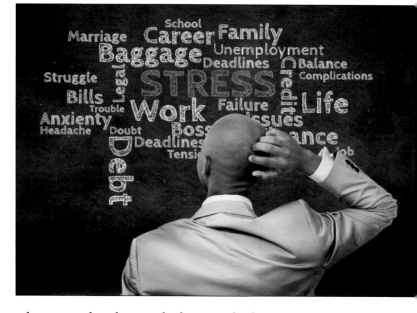

The excess tension through your neck and shoulders might lead to even more pain and headaches. But, before you automatically think these feelings are normal, take the time to observe and understand what your body is trying to communicate. Excess stress is no reason to lay on the couch eating comfort foods full of ingredients that make you sick and gain weight, or to physically abuse yourself with the hardest possible workout without proper progression.

Start listening to your body. Whenever you feel the effects of mental stress, set aside a few minutes to focus on deep diaphragmatic breathing. Move and stretch out what feels tight, restricted, and sore. Deep breathing and mobility work can relieve tension in the entire body so you can enter a clearer state of mind, be better prepared for a workout, and any activities throughout the day. Mindfully breathing through dynamic mobility work is an excellent way to warm up for a workout or any physically challenging task.

The brain is always communicating the present state or status of the body. Millions of proprioceptors throughout the body relay messages to our brain—if we choose to listen to them—while simultaneously controlling the tension and activity of our muscles. The body can quickly evaluate and express feelings of pain, fatigue, sickness, hunger, stress, inflammation, successful integration, overexertion, and injury. Some refer to this as *medical intuition*, which is an awareness of our own physical condition.

If you want to help yourself, start listening to your intuition. Listening to your body can guide you towards taking better care of yourself while understanding what your body needs. Can you relate to any of the following examples of intuition?

EXAMPLE 2:
FEELING WHAT OUR BODIES NEED

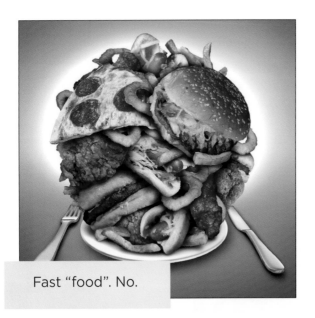

Fast "food". No.

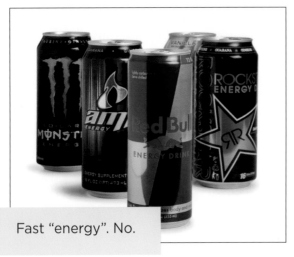

Fast "energy". No.

When we require nourishment, our brains react by triggering hunger and thirst. As soon as feelings of intense hunger set in, we usually crave high calorie foods for immediate energy. For thousands of years, we have associated high calorie meals with replenishing and repairing our bodies. Unfortunately, in modern America, those high calorie meals rarely deliver the nutrients necessary for optimal health.

Have you ever binged on junk food or fast food, stuffing yourself by consuming 1000+ calories at once, only to feel hungry two hours later? That recurrent hunger is the body communicating that it still needs nourishment more than just empty calories.

All foods contain the macronutrients—fat, carbohydrates, and protein—but how many foods contain micronutrients? Junk food, processed food, and fried foods lack vitamins, minerals, natural acids, digestive enzymes, and probiotics. The standard foods in the mainstream American diet severely deprive our bodies of micronutrients.

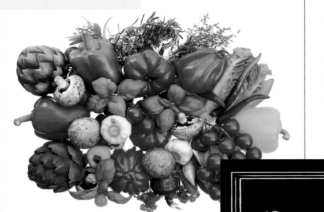

Real food. Yes.

Consequently, without real nourishment, our bodies will send continuous "feed me" and "I'm hungry" signals to the brain. The cravings will continue until the body is nourished by consuming a meal rich in micronutrients. This phenomenon usually contributes to excessive weight gain.

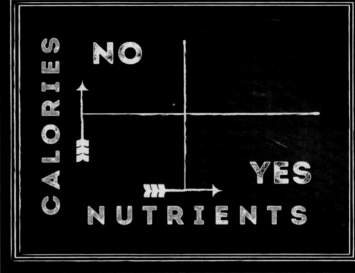

EXAMPLE 3:
FEELING OVERUSE

When we habitually abuse our bodies with excessively strenuous exercise, lack of mental rest, lack of physical sleep, and lack of hydration, we won't feel good very often—except for the few hours after an intense workout while endorphins are active. Exercise should improve your health, longevity, and help you feel good for the activities that make you happy.

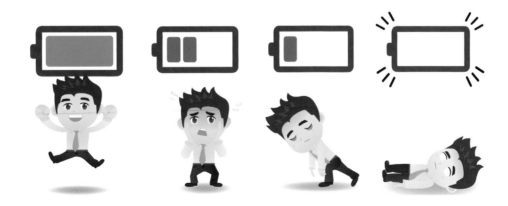

If you have ever suffered from overtraining or excessive muscle soreness, you know exactly what I mean. Without proper recovery, your muscles, tendons, joints, and all your connective tissues will give you a hard time while you are trying to enjoy yourself. When your body gives you warning signs about your current state, be sure to heed them. Overuse injuries such as tendonitis of the shoulder, elbow, knee or ankle, hamstring muscle strains, joint dislocation of the shoulder, and shin splints can usually be avoided.

Did you listen to your body the first time you felt something wrong in the overworked area? Did you notice that the area was tender to the touch, inflamed, or excessively tight? Did you take the time to rest and recover with added nourishment and hydration? Did you massage the irritated area at all? Or did you just think, "NO PAIN NO GAIN" and continue pushing through intense workouts and activities over the next few days or weeks because of a timeline-based goal?

EXAMPLE 4:
WE CAN FEEL MOVEMENT

When throwing a ball, we automatically know if the throw will be good or not—even before we can see where the ball is headed. We inherently know the feeling of efficient body movement. We can feel if our body was fully integrated and efficient. Full body synchronization allows for more powerful and accurate throws with less localized strain on the shoulder and arm. We can see and feel it when we don't get our timing right!

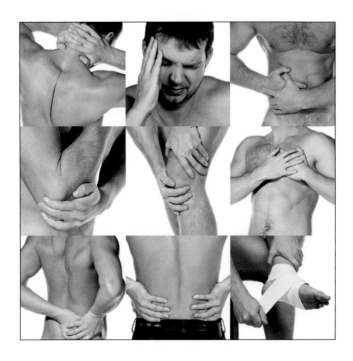

While performing Intrinsic Strength Training® exercises, you can certainly feel if your body is well integrated or not. Successful execution of each IST exercise will require each muscle and joint in the body to synchronize with neighboring muscles and joints. If the weight and exercise are too challenging for you to handle efficiently, the body will let you know! Please pay attention and lower the weight. *When moving feels good and efficient, we feel successful.*

(24) http://www.disabilitycanhappen.org/chances_disability/disability_stats.asp

(25) U.S. Social Security Administration, Disabled Worker Beneficiary Data, December 2012

(26) http://www.ninds.nih.gov/disorders/backpain/detail_backpain.htm

(27) http://www.chekinstitute.com/index.php

(28) Richard G. Carson. J Appl Physiol 101: 1506-1513, 2006. First Published Aug 3, 2006; Doi:10.1152/japplphysiol.00544.2006

(29) Richardson, C., & Hodges, P. (2004). Therapeutic exercise for lumbopelvic stabilization a motor control approach for the treatment and prevention of low back pain (2nd ed.). Edinburgh: Churchill Livingstone.

(30) Hides J A, Stokes M J, Saide M, Jull G A, Cooper D H 1994 Evidence of lumbar multifidus muscle wasting ipsilateral to symptoms in patients with acute/subacute low back pain. Spine 19:165-172

(31) Hides J, Jull G, Richardson C 2000 A clinical palpation test to check the activation of the deep stabilizing muscles of the spine. International Sports Medicine Journal 1:(4)

(32) Gardner-Morse M, Stokes I AF, Lauble JP 1995 Role of the muscles in lumbar spine stability in maximum extension efforts. Journal of Orthopedic Research 12:802-808

(33) Gardner-Morse M G, Stokes I A 1998 The effects of abdominal muscle coactivation on lumbar spine stability. Spine 23:86-91

(34) Stuart McGill. Ultimate Back Fitness and Performance. Backfitpro Inc. (formerly Wabuno Publishers) Waterloo, Ontario, Canada 2009

(35) Medical Dictionary for the Health Professions and Nursing © Farlex 2012 http://medical-dictionary.thefreedictionary.com/motor+learning

(36) The big book of NLP, Shlomo Vaknin

(37) https://en.wikipedia.org/wiki/Posture_%28psychology%29

(38) http://www.ncbi.nlm.nih.gov/pubmed/21877146

(39) http://www.ncbi.nlm.nih.gov/pubmed/15705034

(40) http://www.ncbi.nlm.nih.gov/pubmed/23096062

(41) http://www.acatoday.org/level2_css.cfm?T1ID=13&T2ID=68

(42) Anatomy Trains - Thomas Myers

(43) McCorry, LK (Aug 15, 2007). "Physiology of the autonomic nervous system.". American journal of pharmaceutical education 71 (4): 78. PMID 17786266.

(44) http://informahealthcare.com/doi/pdf/10.3109/17453678909154177

(45) Haid, Regis W. Advances in Spinal Stabilization. Basel: Karger, 2003. Print.

(46) http://jnci.oxfordjournals.org/content/106/7/dju098.full?_ga=1.42982689.527235840.1397574100

(47) http://www.des.umd.edu/os/erg/low.html

(48) http://aje.oxfordjournals.org/content/early/2008/02/25/aje.kwm390.full.pdf

(49) http://aje.oxfordjournals.org/content/167/7/875.full.pdf+html

(50) Leetun DT, Ireland ML, Willson JD, et al. Core stability measures as risk factors for lower extremity injury in athletes. Med Sci Sports Exerc 2004; 36:926–34.

(51) Bergmark A. Stability of the lumbar spine. A study in mechanical engineering. Acta Orthop Scand Suppl 1989; 230:1–54.

(52) Haid, Regis W. Advances in Spinal Stabilization. Basel: Karger, 2003. Print.

(53) Kibler WB, Press J, Sciascia A. The role of core stability in athletic function. Sports Med 2006; 36:189–98.

(54) O McKeon, Patrick. "The Foot Core System: A New Paradigm for Understanding Intrinsic Foot Muscle Function." British Journal of Sports Medicine March (2015). British Journal of Sports Medicine. BMJ Publishing Group. Web. 26 Mar. 2015. http://m.bjsm.bmj.com/content/49/5/290.full

(55) Podiatry Channel, Anatomy of the foot and ankle

(56) Cunningham C, Schilling N, Anders C et al. The influence of foot posture on the cost of transport in humans. J Experimental Biology. 2010; 213:790-797.

(57) Eran Dayan and Leonardo G. Cohen. Neuroplasticity subserving motor skill learning. Neuron November 3rd, 2011; 72 (3): 443-445. NIH Public Access

(58) DeAnna L. Adkins1,2, Jeffery Boychuk1,2, Michael S. Remple3,4, and Jeffrey A. Kleim1,2. Motor training induces experience-specific patterns of plasticity across motor cortex and spinal cord

(59) Kleim. Jeffery A. PhD. Neural Plasticity, Foundation for Neurorehabilitation. TANAS Publishing, 2012!

(60) Blakeslee S, Blakeslee M, The body has a mind of its own, how body maps in your brain help you do (almost) everything better. 2007, Random house trade!

INTRINSIC STRENGTH

TRAINING EXERCISES

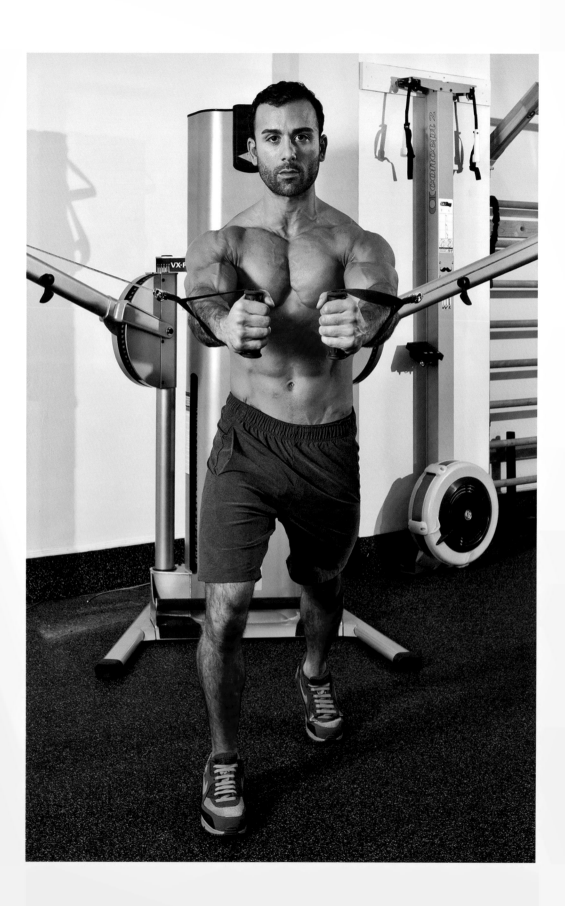

CHEST

Creating a Compatible Chest

Usualy, all forms of the "chest press" are associated with targeting the muscles of the chest. But chest pressing while lying down, and chest pressing while standing are two very different challenges. Have you ever tried pushing a large object like a dresser or couch? Or, have you ever tried to push someone away from you? You feel the tension from these pressing tasks through your whole body, not just your chest and triceps. If pressing and pushing things outside the gym requires the entire body, then why don't we use the entire body while pressing and pushing at the gym?

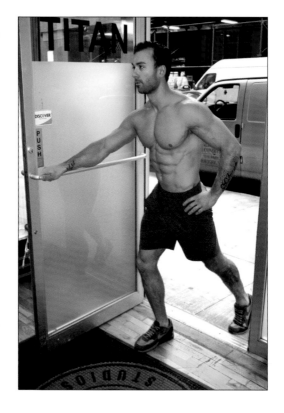

The amount of full body integration and tension are the differences between an IST chest press and a regular chest press. Instead of using a comfy bench for stability, an IST chest press will challenge the entire body with continuous tension from head to toe. Because the lower and upper extremities must work together, core strength becomes essential.

Targeting the chest while incorporating the entire body is the key to developing a symmetrical physique. Preparing yourself and feeling comfortable to push and press while standing up and moving on your feet will unlikely be achieved by seated and lying exercises.

REPLACEMENT EXERCISE FOR
LYING FLAT BENCH CHEST PRESS
IST: FORWARD STEP ONE ARM CHEST PRESS

BOS - bilateral set up position - back facing - alternating forward step
POR - shoulder height - one arm chest press at shoulder height

1. Set up with a bilateral stance with your back facing the resistance point set at shoulder height.
2. Hold one resistance handle with one hand.
3. Perform all three phases of IST with each rep: dynamic acceleration, global repetition, and dynamic deceleration.
4. (Dynamic Acceleration) - Take a step forward—away from the resistance (BOS)— while simultaneously pressing the cable directly in front at shoulder height (POR).
5. (Global Repetition) - Remain in this stance (one foot forward) and execute one complete chest press by bringing the handle into the arm pit then extending the arms outward again. (POR).
6. (Dynamic Deceleration) - Return to the bilateral starting position (BOS) while bringing the resistance (POR) back to the shoulder.
7. Repeat by stepping the opposite foot forward.

ANGELO'S ADVICE

1. Focus on using your entire body for this exercise.
2. Allow the ankles, knees, hips, and shoulders to move as needed for full body muscle activation—but with precise control during each part of the exercise.
3. Actively press the forefoot and big toe of the rear leg into the ground—Activating and stabilizing the entire core to maintain body control, balance, and alignment.
4. Keep your head in a forward-facing, neutral position.

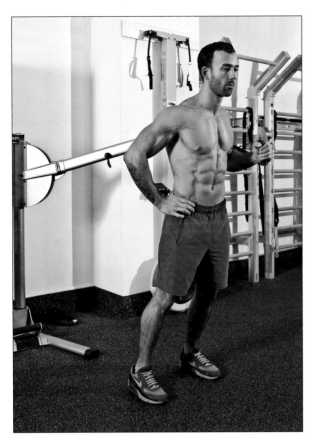
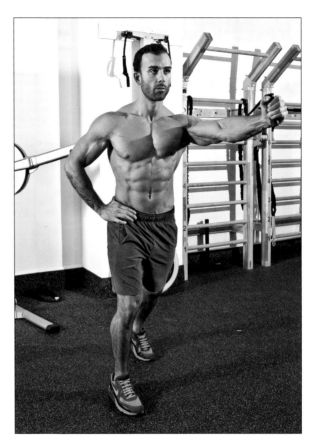

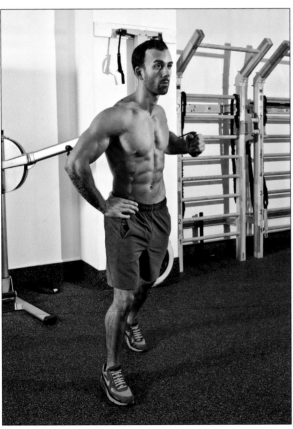
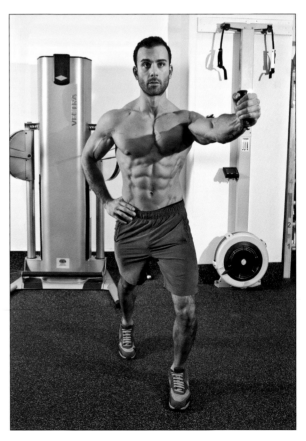

SINGLE ARM (WIDE) VARIATION

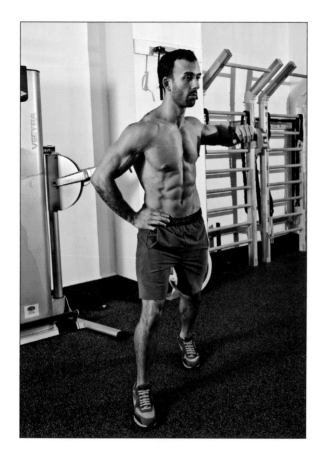 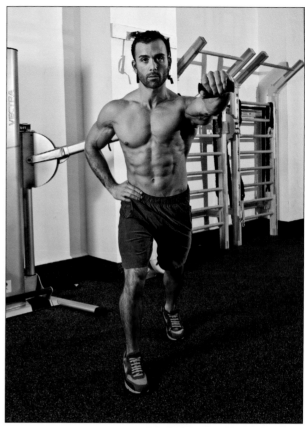

REPLACEMENT EXERCISE FOR
LYING FLAT BENCH CHEST PRESS
IST: SIDE STEP TWO ARM CHEST PRESS

BOS - bilateral set up position - back facing - alternating side step
POR - shoulder height - two arm chest press to shoulder height

1. Set up with a bilateral stance with your back facing the resistance point set at shoulder height.
2. Hold both resistance handles—one in each hand.
3. Perform all three phases of IST with each rep: dynamic acceleration, global repetition, and dynamic deceleration.
4. (Dynamic Acceleration) Take a step to the side—away from the resistance (BOS)—while simultaneously pressing the cable directly in front at shoulder height (POR).
5. (Global Repetition) Remain in this stance (one foot forward) and execute one complete chest press by bringing the handles into the arm pit then extending the arms outward again. (POR).
6. (Dynamic Deceleration) Return to the bilateral starting position (BOS) while bringing the resistance (POR) back to the shoulders.
7. Repeat by stepping the opposite foot to the opposite side.

ANGELO'S ADVICE

1. Focus on using your entire body for this exercise.
2. Allow the ankles, knees, hips, and shoulders to move as needed for full body muscle activation—but with precise control during each part of the exercise.
3. Actively press the forefoot and big toe of the rear leg into the ground—activating and stabilizing the entire core to maintain body control, balance, and alignment.
4. Keep your head in a forward-facing, neutral position.
5. Press the arms out at an angle towards the stepping side.

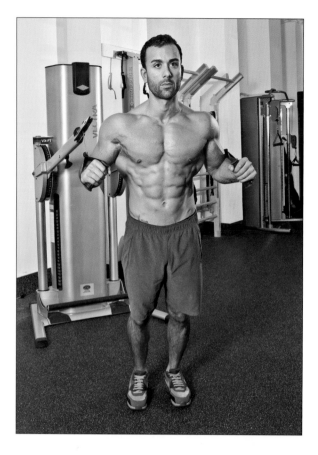
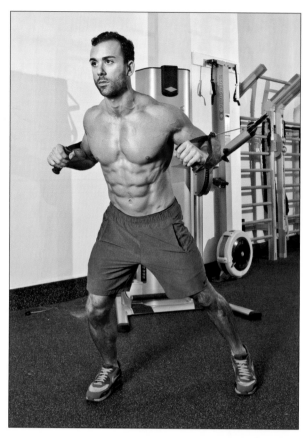
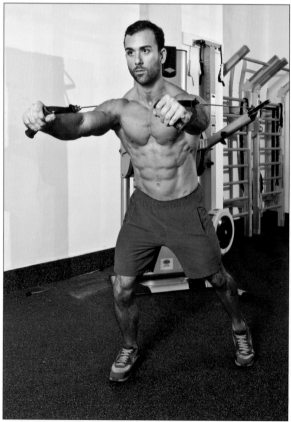
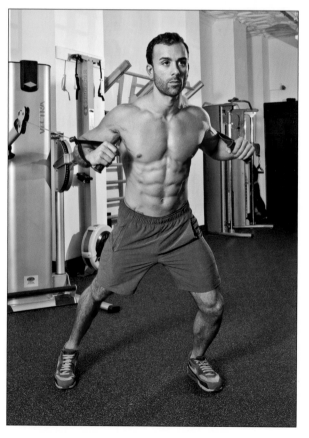

INTRINSIC STRENGTH TRAINING

ONE ARM VARIATION

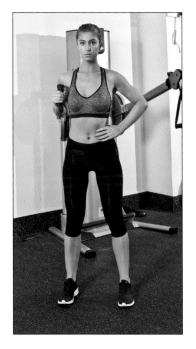 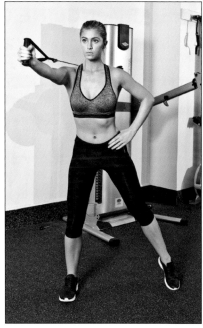 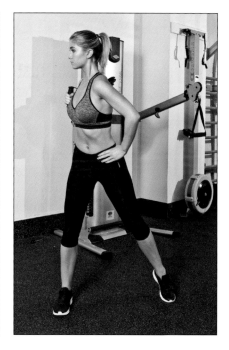

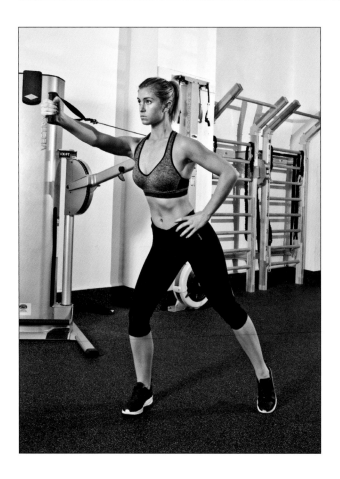 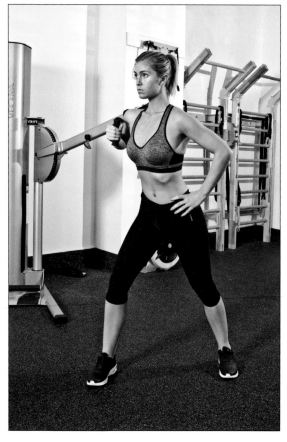

REPLACEMENT EXERCISE FOR
LYING INCLINE CHEST PRESS
IST: FORWARD STEP ONE ARM INCLINE CHEST PRESS

BOS - bilateral set up position - back facing - forward step
POR - hip height - one arm chest press to chin height

1. Set up with a bilateral stance with your back facing the resistance point set at hip height.
2. Hold a resistance handle in one hand.
3. Perform all three phases of IST with each rep: dynamic acceleration, global repetition, and dynamic deceleration.
4. (Dynamic Acceleration) Take a forward step—away from the resistance (BOS)—while simultaneously pressing the cable directly in front at head height (POR).
5. (Global Repetition) Remain in this stance (one foot forward) and execute one complete chest press by bringing the handle into the arm pit then extending the arm outward again (POR).
6. (Dynamic Deceleration) Return to the bilateral starting position (BOS) while bringing the resistance (POR) back to the shoulders.
7. Repeat by stepping the opposite foot forward.

ANGELO'S ADVICE

1. Focus on using your entire body for this exercise.
2. Allow the ankles, knees, hips, and shoulders to move as needed for full body muscle activation —but with precise control during each part of the exercise.
3. Actively press the forefoot and big toe of the rear leg into the ground—activating and stabilizing the entire core to maintain body control, balance, and alignment.
4. Keep your head in a forward-facing, neutral position.

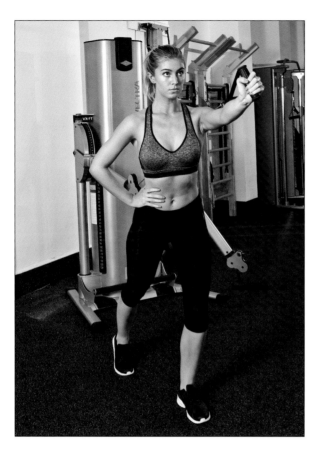
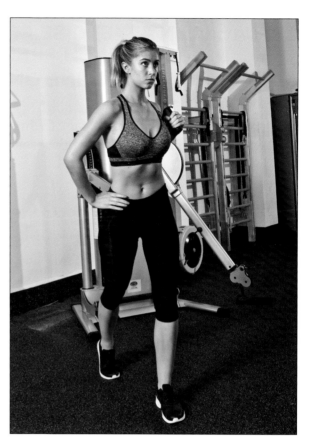
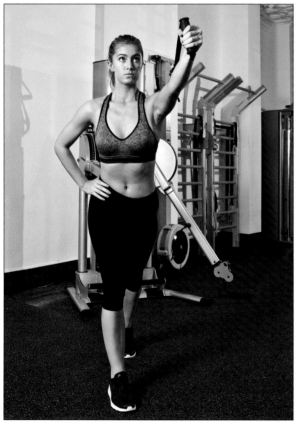
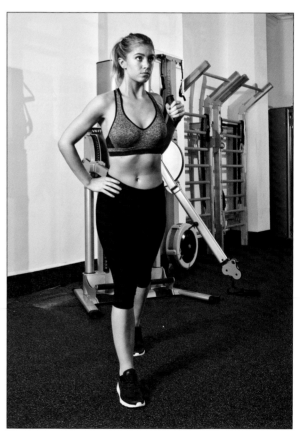

REPLACEMENT EXERCISE FOR
LYING DECLINE BENCH PRESS
IST: REAR STEP DECLINE ONE ARM CHEST PRESS

BOS - bilateral set up position - back facing - alternating rear step
POR - shoulder height - one arm chest press to rib height

1. Set up with a bilateral stance with your back facing the resistance point set at shoulder height.
2. Hold a resistance handle in one hand.
3. Perform all three phases of IST with each rep: dynamic acceleration, global repetition, and dynamic deceleration.
4. (Dynamic Acceleration) Take a rear step—towards from the resistance (BOS)—while simultaneously pressing the cable directly in front at hip height (POR).
5. (Global Repetition) Remain in this stance (one foot forward) and execute one complete chest press by bringing the handle into the arm pit then extending the arm outward again (POR).
6. (Dynamic Deceleration) Return to the bilateral starting position (BOS) while bringing the resistance (POR) back to the shoulders.
7. Repeat by stepping the opposite foot behind you.

ANGELO'S ADVICE

1. Focus on using your entire body for this exercise.
2. Allow the ankles, knees, hips, and shoulders to move as needed for full body muscle activation —but with precise control during each part of the exercise.
3. Actvely press the forefoot and big toe of the rear leg into the ground—activating and stabilizing the entire core to maintain body control, balance, and alignment.
4. Keep your head in a forward-facing, neutral position.

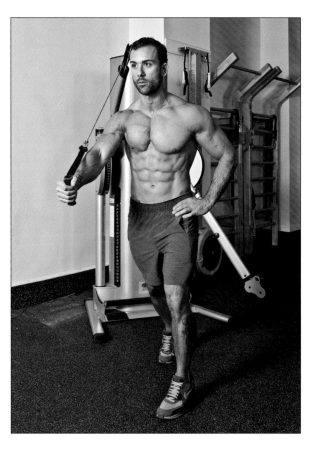
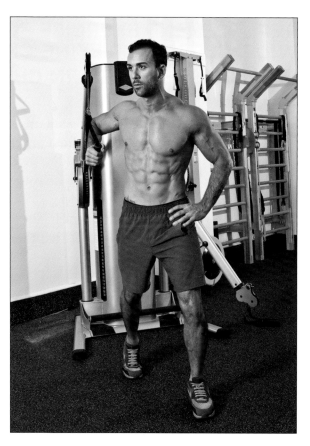
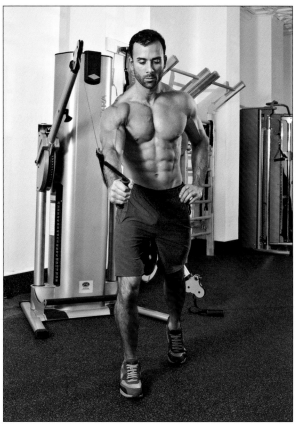
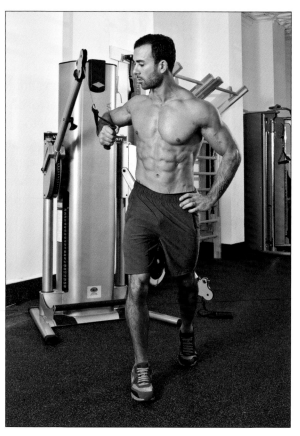

REPLACEMENT EXERCISE FOR
WIDE/CLOSE GRIP LYING CHEST PRESS
IST: SIDE STEP ONE ARM CHEST PRESS ACROSS BODY

BOS - bilateral start position - side set up - side step (side opposite of the resistance point)
POR - shoulder height - one arm chest press across midline to opposite side

1. Set up with a bilateral stance with your back facing the resistance point set at shoulder height.
2. Hold a resistance handle in one hand.
3. Perform all three phases of IST with each rep: dynamic acceleration, global repetition, and dynamic deceleration.
4. (Dynamic Acceleration) Take a side step—away from the resistance (BOS)—while simultaneously pressing the cable directly across the body towards the opposite shoulder at shoulder height (POR).
5. (Global Repetition) Remain in this stance (side step) and execute one complete chest press by bringing the handle into the arm pit then extending the arm outward again. (POR)
6. (Dynamic Deceleration) Return to the bilateral starting position (BOS) while bringing the resistance (POR) back to the shoulders.
7. Repeat by stepping the same foot out to the same side.

ANGELO'S ADVICE

1. Focus on using your entire body for this exercise.
2. Allow the ankles, knees, hips, and shoulders to move as needed for full body muscle activation—but with precise control during each part of the exercise.
3. Actively press the forefoot and big toe of the non stepping leg into the ground—activating and stabilizing the entire core to maintain body control, balance, and alignment.
4. Start by keeping your head in a forward-facing, neutral position.
5. Allow your eyes to follow the resistance handle as you press to ensure core rotation.
6. Repeat for the number of repetitions required by your program.

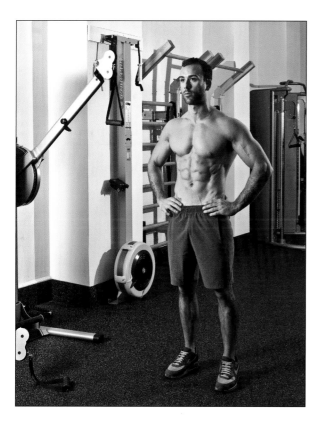
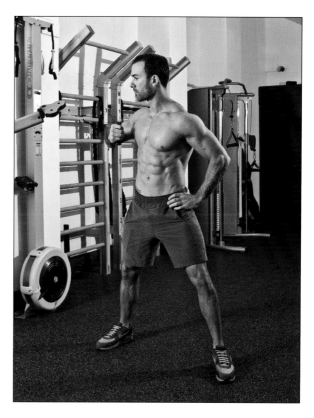
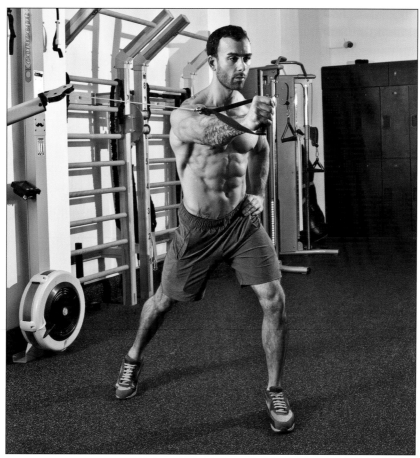

REPLACEMENT EXERCISE FOR
PEC DEC AND CHEST FLY
IST: FORWARD STEP CHEST FLY

BOS - bilateral set up position - side facing the center of both cables' resistance points - alternating forward step

POR - center of both cables' resistance points - hip height - chest fly to shoulder height with full extension

1. Set up with a bilateral stance in-between two resistance points set at shoulder height.
2. Hold both resistance handles - one in each hand.
3. Perform all three phases of IST with each rep: dynamic acceleration, global repetition, and dynamic deceleration.
4. (Dynamic Acceleration) Take a step forward—away from the resistance (BOS)—while simultaneously squeezing the cables directly together in front of you at shoulder height (POR).
5. (Global Repetition) Remain in this stance (one foot forward) and execute one complete chest fly by extending both arms outward (creating a chest stretch) then squeezing the arms back together (POR).
6. (Dynamic Deceleration) Return to the bilateral starting position (BOS) while bringing the resistance (POR) back to the open arm position.
7. Repeat by stepping the opposite foot forward.

ANGELO'S ADVICE

1. Focus on using your entire body for this exercise.
2. Allow the ankles, knees, hips, and shoulders to move as needed for full body muscle activation—but with precise control during each part of the exercise.
3. Actively press the forefoot and big toe of the rear leg into the ground—activating and stabilizing the entire core to maintain body control, balance, and alignment.
4. Keep your head in a forward-facing, neutral position.

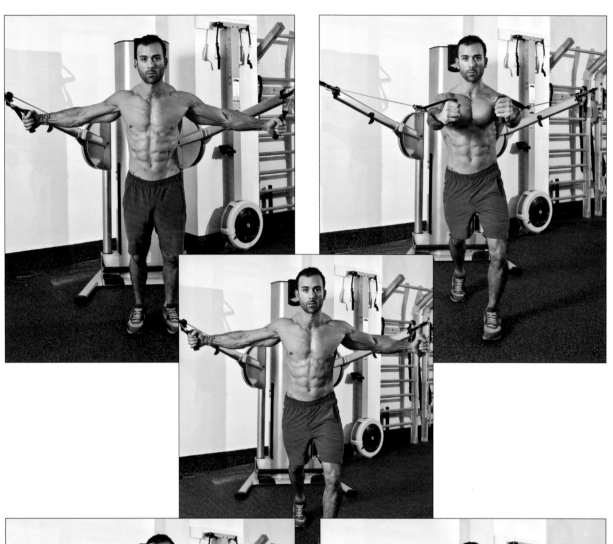
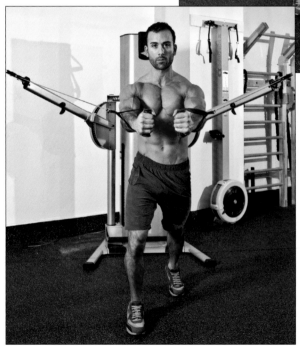
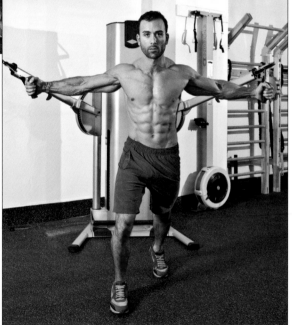

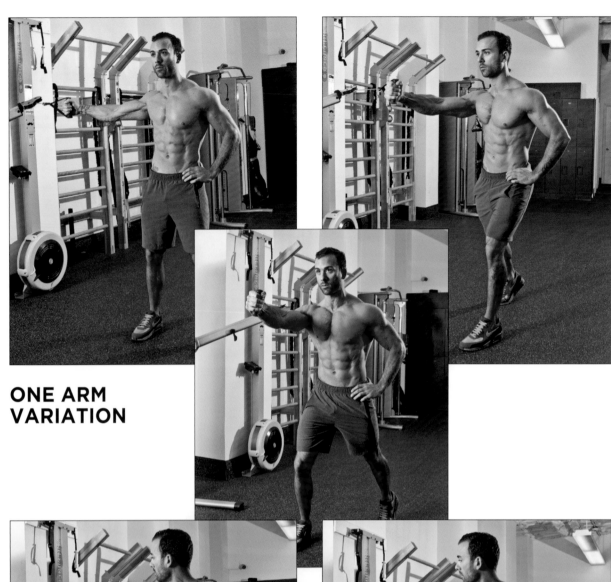

**ONE ARM
VARIATION**

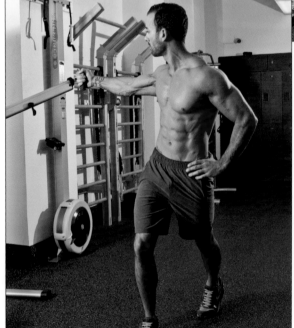

INTRINSIC STRENGTH TRAINING

REPLACEMENT EXERCISE FOR
STANDARD PUSH UP
IST PUSH UP

BOS - bilateral hands and feet - plank position
POR - pushup - global rotation - eye gaze over alternating shoulders at bottom of push up
   (concentric contraction)

1. Start with your feet in a bilateral stance, shoulder width apart.
2. Walk both hands out on the floor until you are in a plank position.
3. Do a regular push up, then begin a second push up.
4. At the bottom of the second push up, gaze over the back of your right shoulder.
5. Complete a third push up, and gaze over the back of the left shoulder at the bottom of the rep.
6. Perform a series of three push ups to complete one repetition of an IST push up.
   a. First push up: look over the right shoulder.
   b. Second push up: look between your hands.
   c. Third push up: look over left shoulder.

ANGELO'S ADVICE

1. Your eyes will direct your head, shoulders, spine, and hips to rotate towards the same side as focal point (looking above the shoulder).
2. Your eyes will direct your head, shoulders, spine, and hips to rotate towards the same focal point (above the shoulder).
3. Actively apply pressure into the ground through your legs and feet to create lower body tension.
4. Actively apply pressure into the ground through your shoulders and fingers to create upper body tension.
5. This extremity tension will radiate through the core - ensuring core tension and more muscular activation.

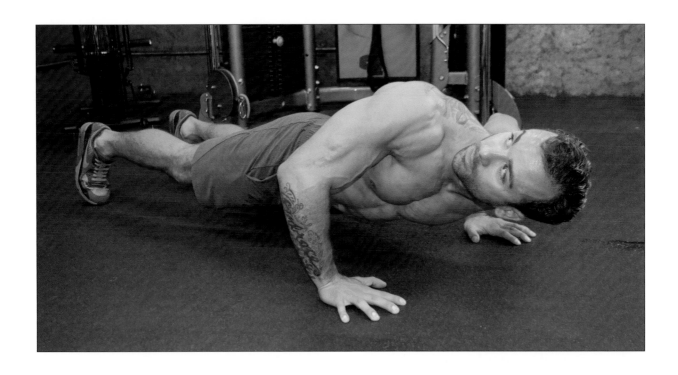

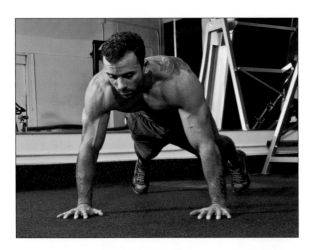

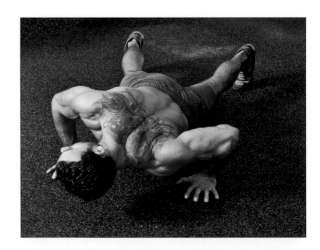

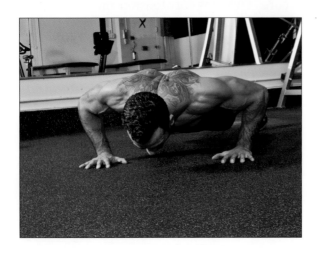

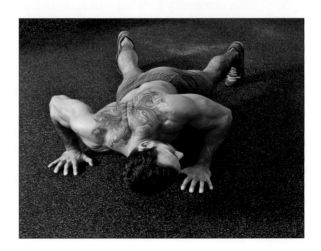

INTRINSIC STRENGTH TRAINING

Back Beneficial Workout

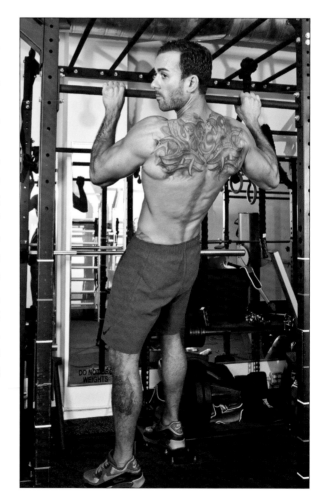

During a back-beneficial workout, you will pull yourself towards something, or pull something towards yourself. In both cases, you will immediately feel your core engage. Unfortunately, conventional fitness training avoids training the core and lower extremities while building a muscular back. Performing pushing or pulling exercises while sitting completely takes the core out of the equation—even though the back is a large part of the core. Connective tissue (thoracolumbar fascia) joins the big muscles of the back with the hip, spine, and ribs. This interconnected tissue provides a foundation which protects the spine and supports the upper and lower extremities, especially when they move. A strong, efficient back requires a strong, efficient core. You can build a back that's beneficial to your real life outside the gym by training in dynamic upright positions.

REPLACEMENT EXERCISE FOR SEATED ROW
IST: SIDE STEP ROW

BOS - bilateral starting position - forward facing - alternating side step
POR - shoulder height - one arm row at shoulder height

1. Set up with a bilateral stance while facing the resistance point set at shoulder height.
2. Hold one resistance handle with one hand.
3. Perform all three phases of IST with each rep: dynamic acceleration, global repetition, and dynamic deceleration.
4. (Dynamic Acceleration) Take a step to the side—away from the resistance (BOS)— while simultaneously pulling the cable directly into the shoulder (POR).
5. (Global Repetition) Remain in this stance (one foot to the side) and execute one complete row by extending the arm outward at shoulder height and back into the arm pit (POR).
6. (Dynamic Deceleration) Return to the bilateral starting position (BOS) while bringing the resistance (POR) back out at the shoulder.
7. Repeat by stepping the opposite foot to the opposite side.

ANGELO'S ADVICE

1. Focus on using your entire body for this exercise.
2. Allow the ankles, knees, hips, and shoulders to move as needed for full body muscle activation—but with precise control during each part of the exercise.
3. Actively press the forefoot and big toe of the non stepping leg into the ground—activating and stabilizing the entire core to maintain body control, balance, and alignment.
4. Keep your head in a forward-facing, neutral position.
5. Allow the side step to change the angle of the rowing arms - involving different muscle fibers.

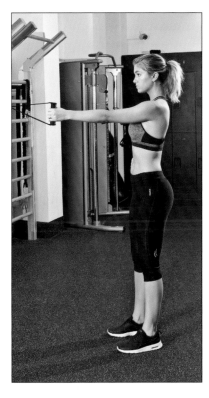
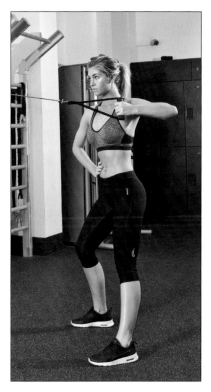
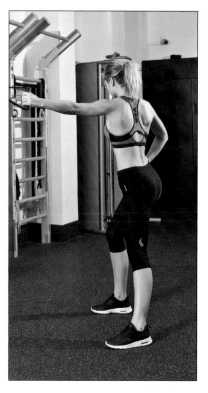
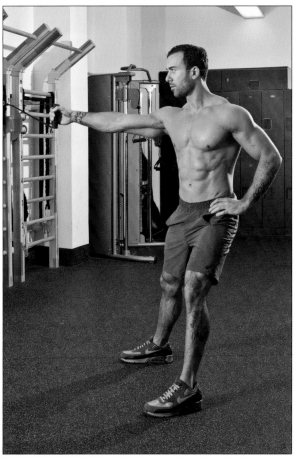
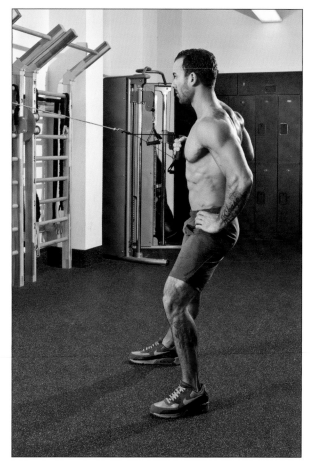

TWO ARM VARIATION

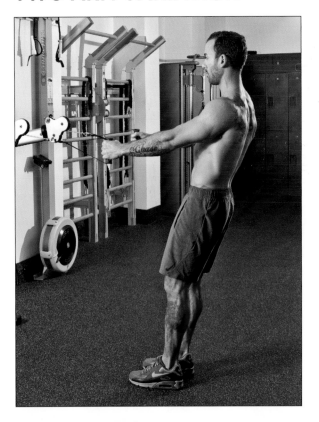
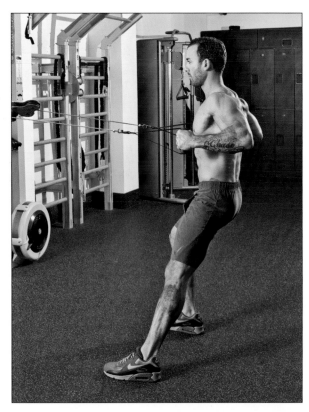
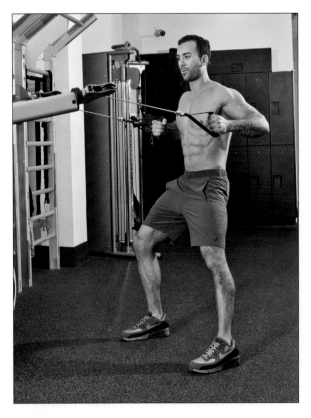
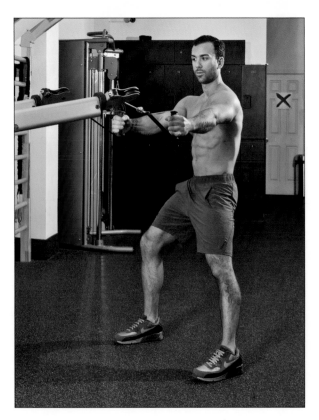

REPLACEMENT EXERCISE FOR
SEATED ROW
IST: REAR STEP ROW

BOS - bilateral starting position - forward facing - alternating rear step
POR - pelvis height - one arm row at shoulder height

1. Set up with a bilateral stance while facing the resistance point set at pelvis height.
2. Hold one resistance handle with one hand.
3. Perform all three phases of IST with each rep: dynamic acceleration, global repetition, and dynamic deceleration.
4. (Dynamic Acceleration) Take a step behind—away from the resistance (BOS)—while simultaneously pulling the cable directly into the shoulder (POR).
5. (Global Repetition) Remain in this stance (one foot in a rear step) and execute one complete row by extending the arm outward at shoulder height and back into the arm pit (POR).
6. (Dynamic Deceleration) Return to the bilateral starting position (BOS) while bringing the resistance (POR) back out at the shoulder.
7. Repeat by stepping the opposite foot to the rear.

ANGELO'S ADVICE

1. Focus on using your entire body for this exercise.
2. Allow the ankles, knees, hips, and shoulders to move as needed for full body muscle activation—but with precise control during each part of the exercise.
3. Actively press the forefoot and big toe of the non stepping leg into the ground—activating and stabilizing the entire core to maintain body control, balance, and alignment.
4. Keep your head in a forward-facing, neutral position.

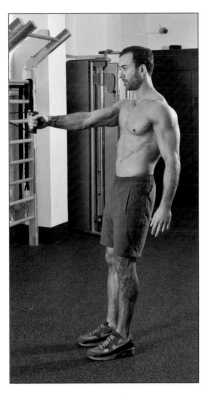
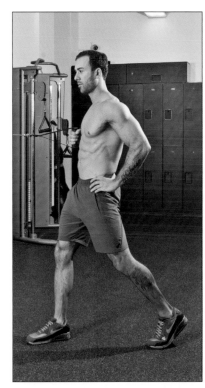
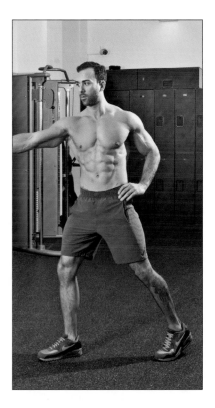

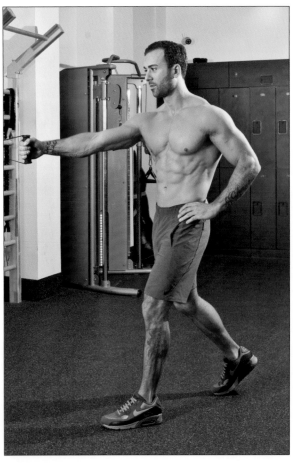
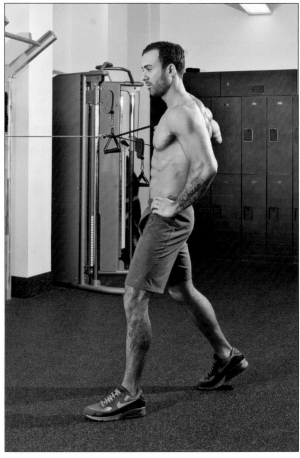

INTRINSIC STRENGTH TRAINING

HEIGHT VARIATION

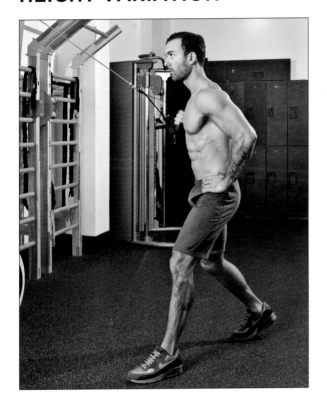 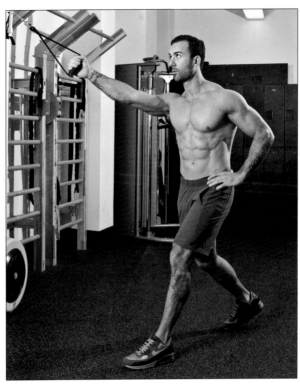

TWO ARM VERSION

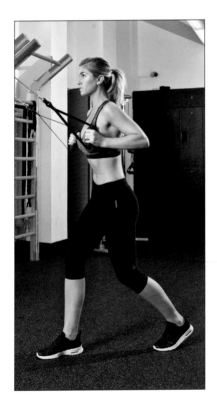 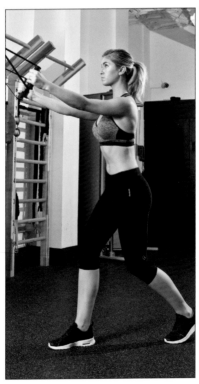 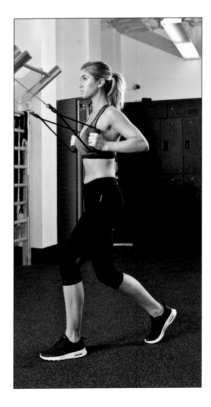

REPLACEMENT EXERCISE FOR SEATED ROW
IST: REAR CROSSOVER STEP ROW

BOS - bilateral starting position - forward facing - alternating rear crossover step
POR - pelvis height - one arm row to shoulder

1. Set up with a bilateral stance while facing the resistance point set at pelvis height.
2. Hold one resistance handle with one hand.
3. Perform all three phases of IST with each rep: dynamic acceleration, global repetition, and dynamic deceleration.
4. (Dynamic Acceleration) Take a rear cross over step to the opposite side—away from the resistance (BOS)—while simultaneously pulling the cable directly into the shoulder (POR).
5. (Global Repetition) Remain in this stance (one foot in a rear cross over step) and execute one complete row by extending the arm outward at shoulder height and back into the arm pit (POR).
6. (Dynamic Deceleration) Return to the bilateral starting position (BOS) while bringing the resistance (POR) back out at the shoulder.
7. Repeat by stepping the opposite foot behind the opposite side.

ANGELO'S ADVICE

1. Focus on using your entire body for this exercise.
2. Allow the ankles, knees, hips, and shoulders to move as needed for full body muscle activation—but with precise control during each part of the exercise.
3. Actively press the forefoot and big toe of the non stepping leg into the ground—activating and stabilizing the entire core to maintain body control, balance, and alignment.
4. Keep your head in a forward-facing, neutral position.

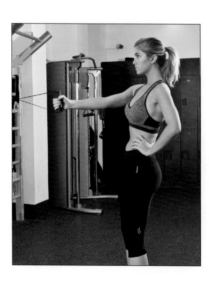 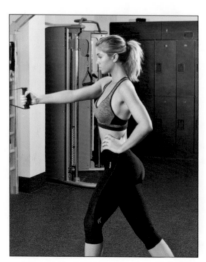 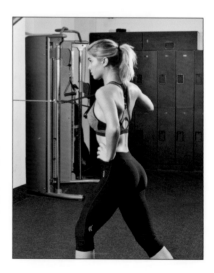

INTRINSIC STRENGTH TRAINING

TWO ARM VARIATION

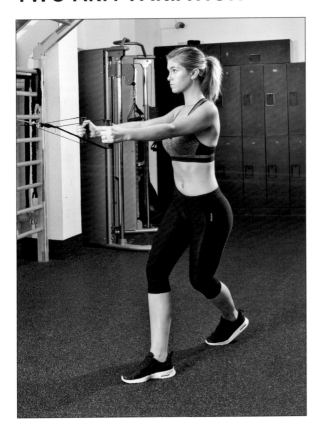
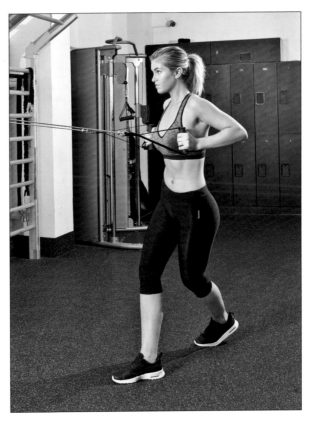
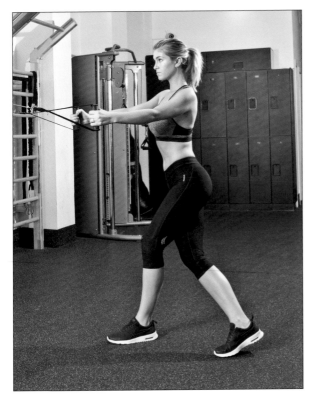
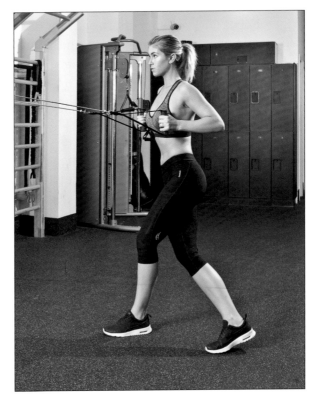

REPLACEMENT EXERCISE FOR SEATED ROW
IST: REAR ROTATIONAL STEP ROW

BOS - bilateral starting position - forward facing - rear rotation step - same side as resistance
POR - shoulder height - one arm row to shoulder

1. Set up with a bilateral stance while facing the resistance point set at shoulder height.
2. Hold one resistance handle with one hand.
3. Perform all three phases of IST with each rep: dynamic acceleration, global repetition, and dynamic deceleration.
4. (Dynamic Acceleration) Take a rear rotation step with the same side as resistance handle—away from the resistance (BOS)—while simultaneously pulling the cable directly into the shoulder (POR).
5. (Global Repetition) Remain in this stance (one foot rear rotated) and execute one complete row by extending the arm outward at shoulder height and back into the arm pit. (POR)
6. (Dynamic Deceleration) Return to the bilateral starting position (BOS) while bringing the resistance (POR) back out at the shoulder.
7. Repeat for the number of repetitions required by your program.

ANGELO'S ADVICE

1. Focus on using your entire body for this exercise.
2. Allow the ankles, knees, hips, and shoulders to move as needed for full body muscle activation—but with precise control during each part of the exercise.
3. Actively press the forefoot and big toe of the non stepping leg into the ground—activating and stabilizing the entire core to maintain body control, balance, and alignment.
4. Keep your head in a forward-facing, neutral position.
5. Allow your eyes to follow the resistance handle as you row to ensure core rotation.
6. Be sure the elbow is at shoulder height during the row to ensure proper activation of the upper back and shoulder musculature.

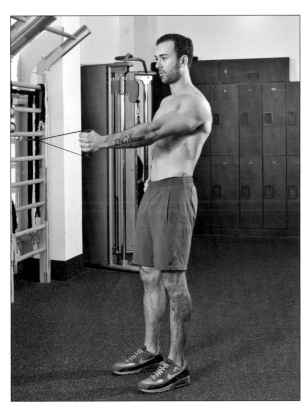
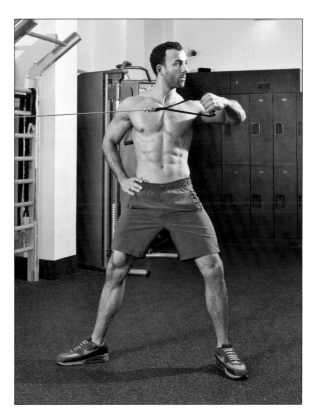
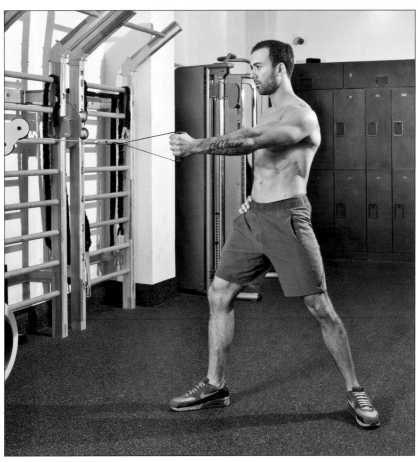

REPLACEMENT EXERCISE FOR
SEATED ROW
IST: FORWARD STEP ROW

BOS - bilateral starting position - forward facing - forward step - alternating
POR - ankle height - one arm row at shoulder

1. Set up with a bilateral stance, facing the resistance point at ankle height.
2. Hold a resistance handle with one hand and pull into the arm pit to start.
3. Perform all three phases of IST with each rep: dynamic acceleration, global repetition, and dynamic deceleration.
4. Take a forward step towards the resistance, while simultaneously letting the arm extend out from the arm pit (BOS+POR).
5. Remain in this stance (rear rotation step) and execute one complete row by bringing the handle into the arm pit, then extending the arm outward again.
6. Return to the starting position under control by simultaneously stepping back to the bilateral stance (BOS) and bringing the resistance point (POR) back to the arm pit.

ANGELO'S ADVICE

1. Focus on using your entire body for this exercise.
2. Actively press the forefoot and big toe of the stepping leg into the ground to activate and stabilize the entire core to keep in control of the body's balance.
3. Allow the ankles, knees, hips, and shoulders to move as needed—but with precise control during each part of the exercise for full body muscle activation.
4. Keep your head in a forward-facing, neutral position.
5. Keep your eyes on the resistance handle as you press to ensure core rotation.
6. Repeat for the number of repetitions required by your program.

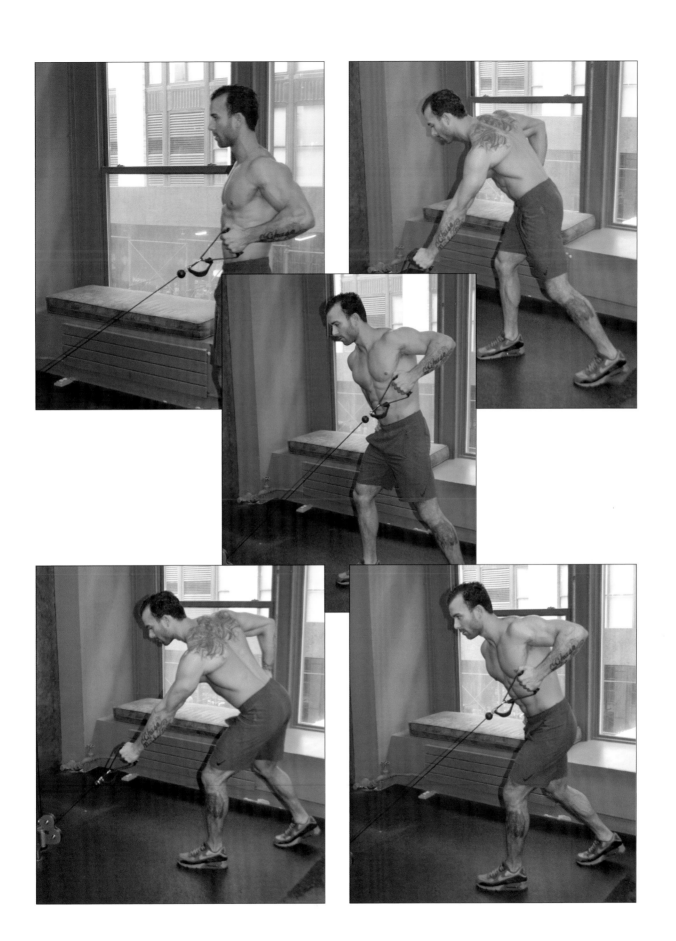

REPLACEMENT EXERCISE FOR
LAT PULL DOWN
IST: REAR STEP PULL DOWN

BOS - bilateral set up position - forward facing - alternating rear step
POR - overhead height - one arm pull down to arm pit

1. Set up with a bilateral stance, facing the resistance point at overhead height.
2. Hold a resistance handle with one hand.
3. Perform all three phases of IST with each rep: dynamic acceleration, global repetition, and dynamic deceleration.
4. Take a rear step away from the resistance, while simultaneously pulling the arm to the arm pit (BOS+POR).
5. Remain in this stance (rear step) and execute one complete row by extending the arm outward again and pulling back to the armpit.
6. Return to the starting position under control by simultaneously stepping back to the bilateral stance (BOS) and extending the arm back towards the resistance point (POR).

ANGELO'S ADVICE

1. Focus on using your entire body for this exercise.
2. Actively press the forefoot and big toe of the non stepping leg into the ground to activate and stabilize the entire core to keep in control of the body's balance.
3. Allow the ankles, knees, hips, and shoulders to move as needed—but with precise control during each part of the exercise for full body muscle activation.
4. Keep your head in a forward-facing, neutral position.
5. Repeat by stepping the opposite foot behind you.

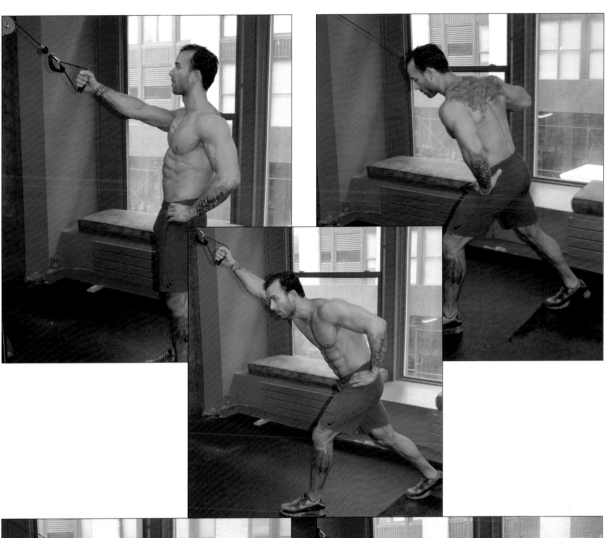
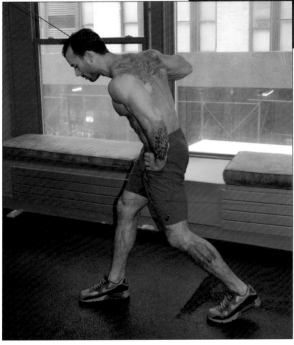
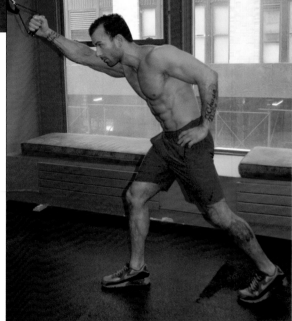

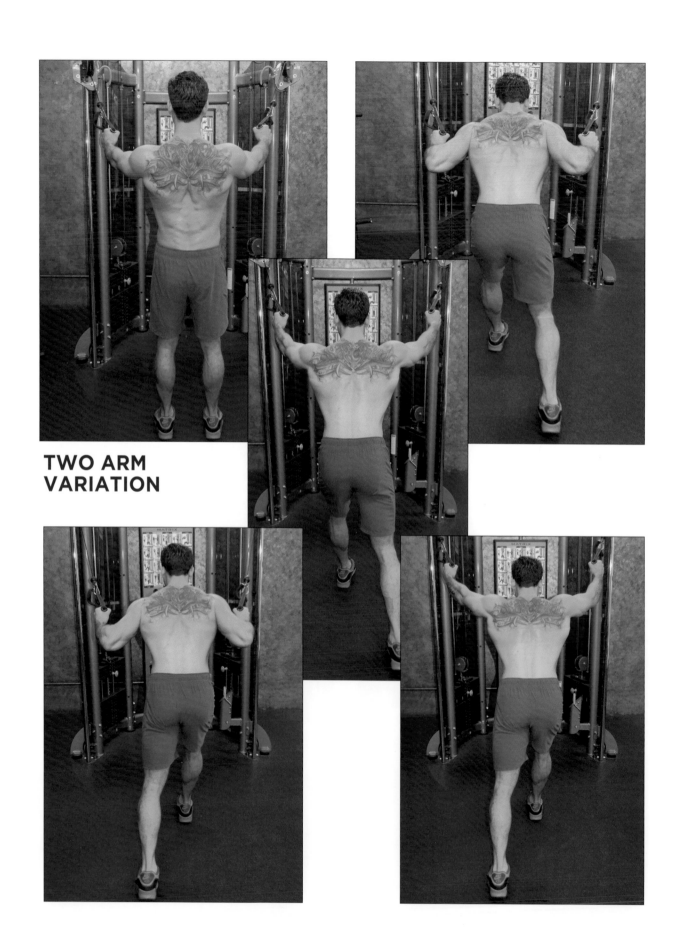

TWO ARM
VARIATION

INTRINSIC STRENGTH TRAINING

REPLACEMENT EXERCISE FOR
STRAIGHT ARM PULL DOWN
IST: REAR CROSSOVER STEP STRAIGHT ARM PULL

BOS - bilateral start position - side facing - rear crossover step
POR - overhead cable - one arm pull down towards pelvis

1. Set up with a bilateral stance, side facing the resistance point at overhead height.
2. Hold a resistance handle with one hand—using arm closest to the (POR).
3. Perform all three phases of IST with each rep: dynamic acceleration, global repetition, and dynamic deceleration.
4. Take a rear cross over step away from the resistance, (with the foot closest to POR) while simultaneously pulling the arm to the arm pit (straight arm, not bent) (BOS+POR).
5. Remain in this stance (rear cross over step) and execute one complete pull by raising the arm overhead and pulling it back to the pelvis.
6. Return to the starting position under control by simultaneously stepping back to the bilateral stance (BOS) and extending the arm back towards the resistance point (POR).

ANGELO'S ADVICE

1. Focus on using your entire body for this exercise.
2. Actively press the forefoot and big toe of the non stepping leg into the ground to activate and stabilize the entire core to keep in control of the body's balance.
3. Allow the ankles, knees, hips, and shoulders to move as needed—but with precise control during each part of the exercise for full body muscle activation.
4. Keep your head in a forward-facing, neutral position.
5. Repeat for the number of repetitions required by your program.

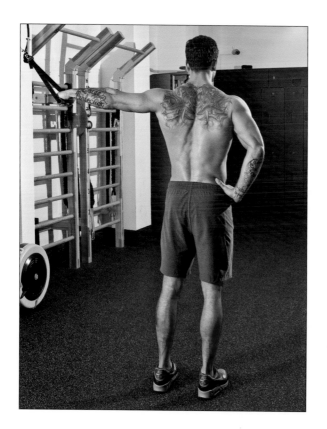

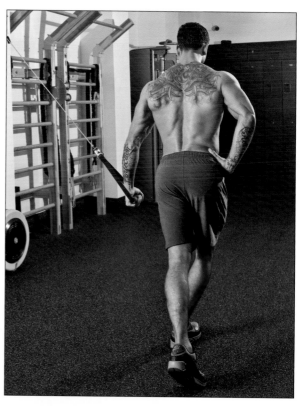

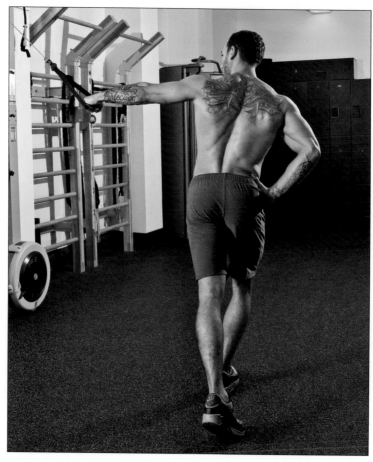

INTRINSIC STRENGTH TRAINING

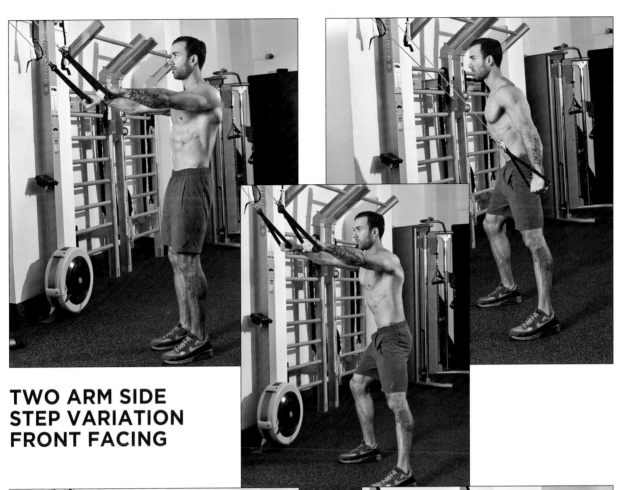

TWO ARM SIDE STEP VARIATION FRONT FACING

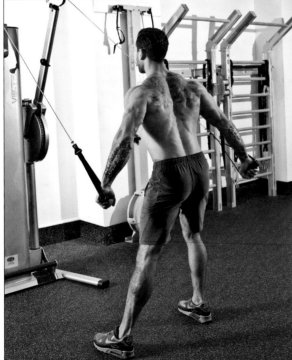

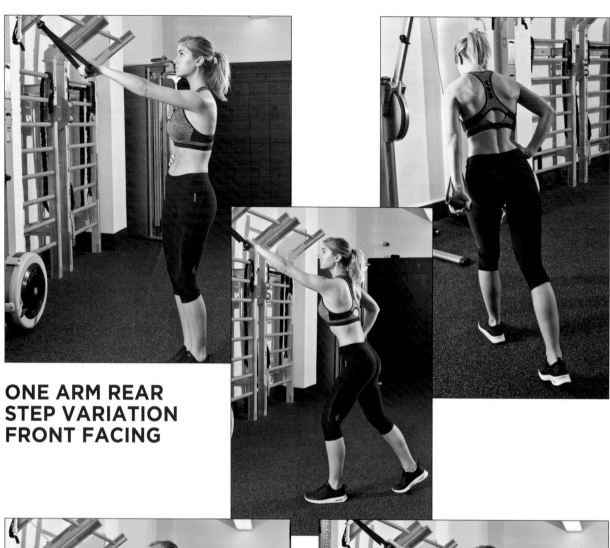

ONE ARM REAR
STEP VARIATION
FRONT FACING

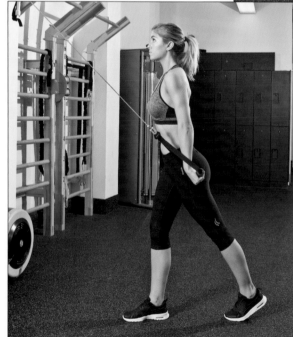

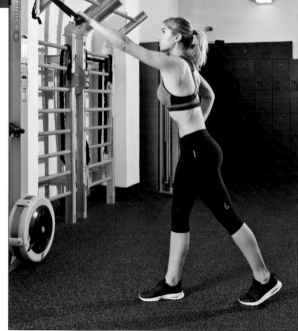

INTRINSIC STRENGTH TRAINING

REPLACEMENT EXERCISE FOR BENT-OVER ROW
IST: FORWARD STEP BELLY ROW

BOS - bilateral start position - forward facing - alternating forward step
POR - weight held at pelvis - belly row

1. Set up with a bilateral stance while holding a barbell / hand weight at pelvis height with one or two hands.
2. Perform all three phases of IST with each rep: dynamic acceleration, global repetition, and dynamic deceleration.
3. (Dynamic Acceleration) Take a forward step away from the start position (BOS)—while simultaneously extending the arms straight towards the ground, directly underneath the shoulder.(POR).
4. (Global Repetition) Remain in this stance (forward step) and execute one complete row by pulling the arms to the center of the belly and extend back out underneath the shoulder (POR).
5. (Dynamic Deceleration) Return back to the bilateral starting position (BOS) while bringing the resistance (POR) back to pelvis height.
6. Repeat by stepping forward with the opposite foot.

ANGELO'S ADVICE

1. Focus on using your entire body for this exercise.
2. Allow the ankles, knees, hips, and shoulders to move as needed for full body muscle activation—but with precise control during each part of the exercise.
3. Actively press the forefoot and big toe of the stepping leg into the ground—activating and stabilizing the entire core to maintain body control, balance, and alignment.
4. Be sure to keep a strong and erect posture by applying tension throughout the core, keeping the spine in an neutral position. Keep your head in a forward-facing, neutral position.

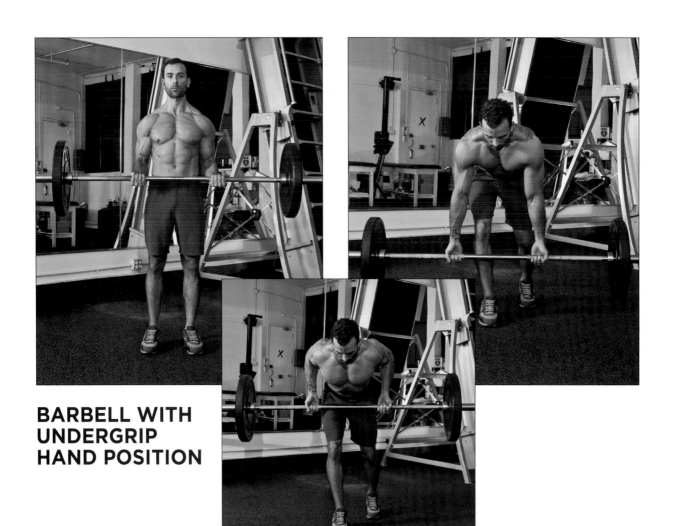

BARBELL WITH UNDERGRIP HAND POSITION

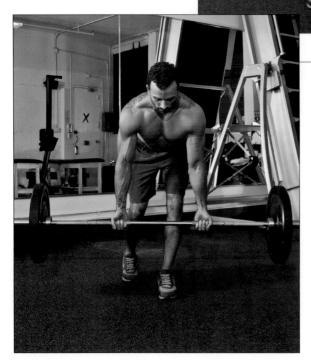

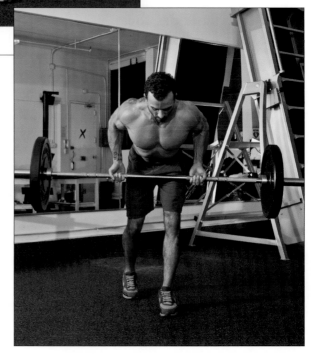

REPLACEMENT EXERCISE FOR BENT-OVER ROW
IST: REAR STEP BELLY ROW (TWO HAND WEIGHTS)

BOS - bilateral start position - alternating rear step
POR - forward facing - holding weight at pelvis - floor to belly row

1. Same as above, repeat with an alternating step backwards.

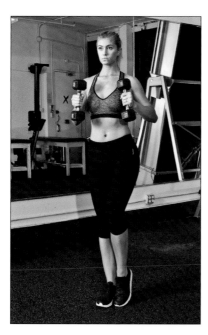 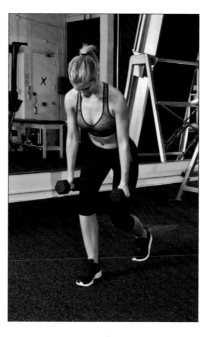 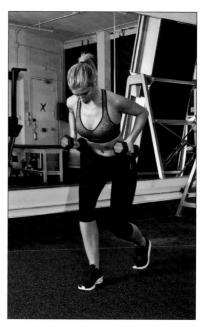

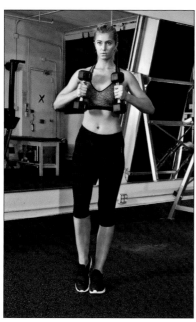 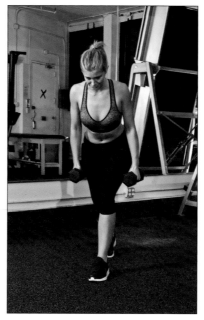 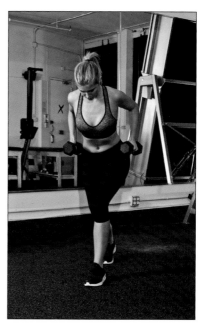

REPLACEMENT EXERCISE FOR BENT-OVER ROW
IST: REAR ROTATION STEP BELLY ROW (MEDICINE BALL)

BOS - bilateral start position - alternating rear rotation step
POR - forward facing - hold weight at pelvis - floor to belly row

1.   Same as above, repeat with alternating rear rotation step.

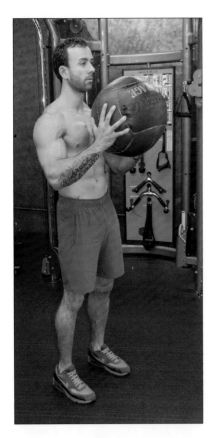
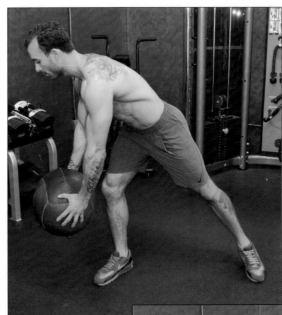

REPLACEMENT EXERCISE FOR
BENT-OVER ROW
IST: SIDE STEP BELLY ROW (TWO HAND WEIGHTS)

BOS - bilateral start position - alternating side step
POR - forward facing - hold weight at pelvis - floor to belly row

1. Same as above, repeat with alternating side step.

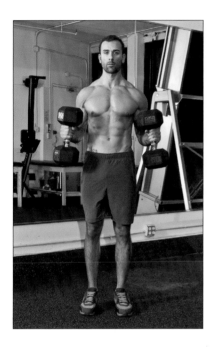 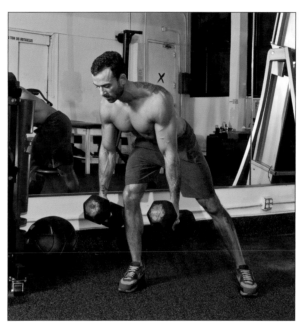

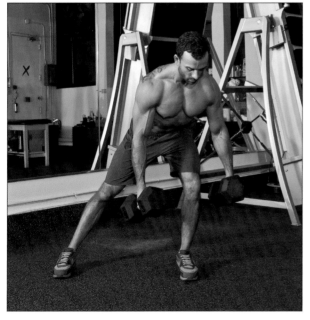 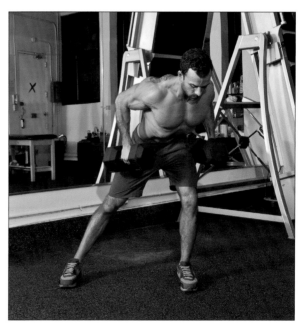

REPLACEMENT EXERCISE FOR STANDARD PULL UP
IST PULL UP

BOS - both hands on pull up bar or gymnastic rings - hanging from overhead
POR - pull up - global rotation - gaze over and behind the shoulder at the top
of concentric contraction

1. Grasp a pull up bar with your hands and arms shoulder width apart.
2. Complete a regular pull up.
   Complete a second pull up, but at the top of the bar, gaze over the back of the right shoulder.
3. Complete a third pull up, and at the top of the bar, gaze over the back of the left shoulder.
4. Perform a series of three pull ups to complete one repetition of IST pull ups.
   a. First pull up: look over the right shoulder.
   b. Second pull up; look between hands or straight ahead.
   c. Third pull up: look over left shoulder.

ANGELO'S ADVICE

1. Allow every joint to help with the full body rotation.
2. Your eyes will direct your head, shoulders, spine, and hips to rotate towards the same side as focal point (looking behind the shoulder).
3. Actively apply pressure into the bar through your shoulders and fingers to create more tension to radiate through the upper body into the core.

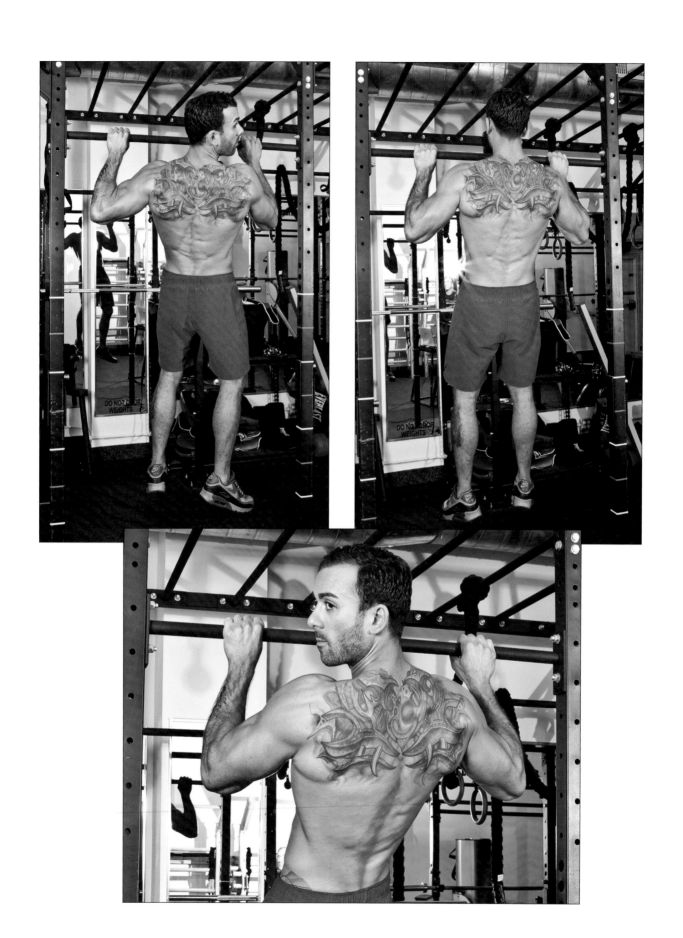

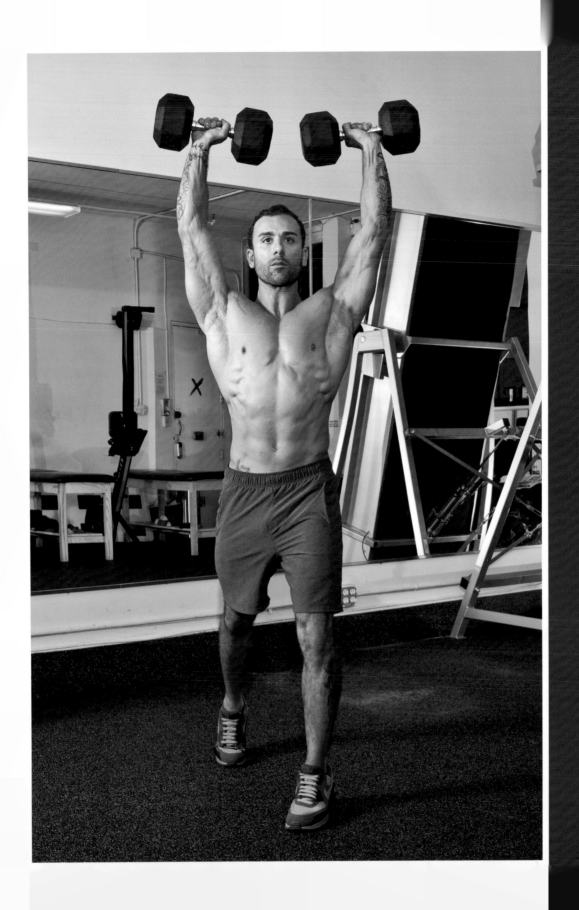

SHOULDERS

Symmetrical Shoulders

For the arms to reach in every direction, the shoulders are some of the most mobile joints in the body. Shoulders are required to control and stabilize every movement of the arms while maintaining a safe position relative to the surrounding joints. When we reach for something to our side, the entire body rotates in that same direction. The action of the arms will change the orientation of the shoulders, which will effect the alignment of all the other joints and muscles in the body. A seated or stationary approach to shoulder training will limit your shoulders' abilities and longevity. Training from all angles with dynamic body positions is essential to the success of ALL shoulders.

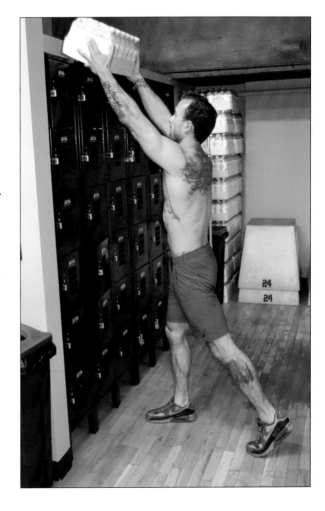

REPLACEMENT EXERCISE FOR SHOULDER/MILITARY PRESS
IST: FORWARD STEP SHOULDER PRESS

BOS - bilateral start position - alternating forward step
POR - shoulder height - front rack position - one arm shoulder press forward

1. Set up with a bilateral stance while holding a hand weight at shoulder height with one hand.
2. Perform all three phases of IST with each rep: dynamic acceleration, global repetition, and dynamic deceleration.
3. (Dynamic Acceleration) Take a forward step away from the start position (BOS)—while simultaneously pressing the arm directly upward above the shoulder. (POR)
4. (Global Repetition) Remain in this stance (forward step) and execute one complete shoulder press by pulling the arm back to the sternum at shoulder height and extend directly above the shoulder (POR).
5. (Dynamic Deceleration) Return back to the bilateral starting position (BOS) while bringing the resistance (POR) back to shoulder height.
6. Repeat by stepping forward with the opposite foot.

ANGELO'S ADVICE

1. Focus on using your entire body for this exercise.
2. Allow the ankles, knees, hips, and shoulders to move as needed for full body muscle activation—but with precise control during each part of the exercise.
3. Actively press the forefoot and big toe of the rear leg into the ground—activating and stabilizing the entire core to maintain body control, balance, and alignment.
4. Keep your head in a forward-facing, neutral position.

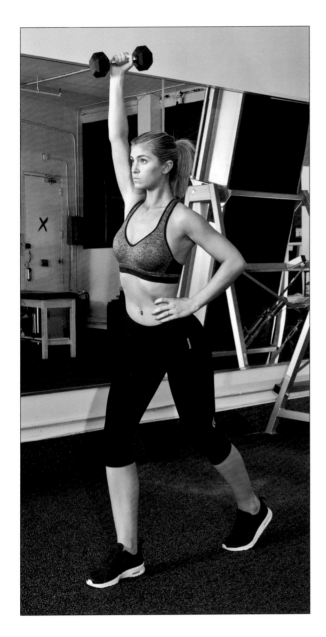
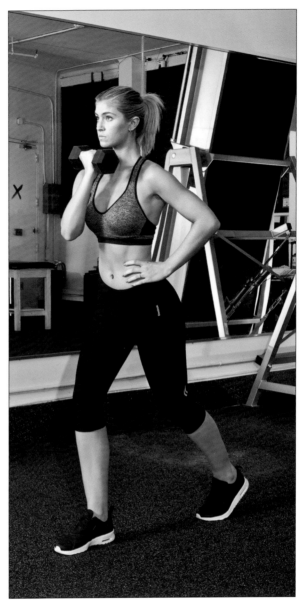

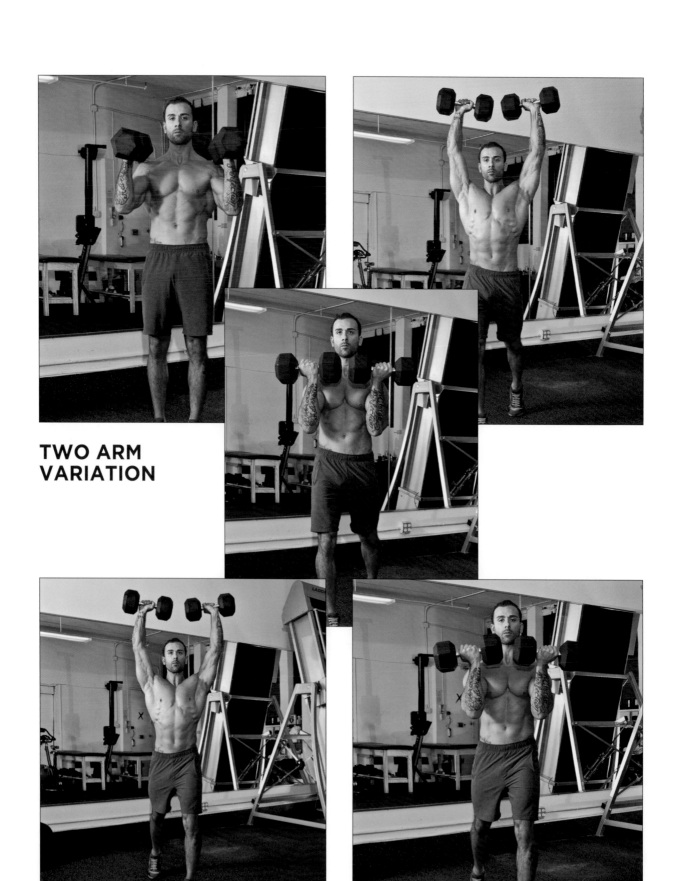

TWO ARM
VARIATION

INTRINSIC STRENGTH TRAINING

REPLACEMENT EXERCISE FOR SHOULDER/MILITARY PRESS
IST: SIDE STEP OVERHEAD PRESS

BOS - bilateral start position - side facing - side step (with the foot furthest from the resistance, stepping away from the resistance.

POR - pelvis height cable or Shoulder height hand weight - one arm shoulder press overhead towards midline

1. Set up with a bilateral stance while holding a hand weight at shoulder height with one hand.
2. Perform all three phases of IST with each rep: dynamic acceleration, global repetition, and dynamic deceleration.
3. (Dynamic Acceleration) Take a side step away from the start position (BOS)—while simultaneously pressing the arm directly upward above the shoulder. (POR)
4. (Global Repetition) Remain in this stance (side step) and execute one complete shoulder press by pulling the arm back to the sternum at shoulder height and extend directly above the shoulder (POR).
5. (Dynamic Deceleration) Return back to the bilateral starting position (BOS) while bringing the resistance (POR) back to shoulder height
6. Repeat by stepping to the opposite side with the opposite foot.

ANGELO'S ADVICE

1. Focus on using your entire body for this exercise.
2. Allow the ankles, knees, hips, and shoulders to move as needed for full body muscle activation—but with precise control during each part of the exercise.
3. Actively press the forefoot and big toe of the non stepping leg into the ground—activating and stabilizing the entire core to maintain body control, balance, and alignment.

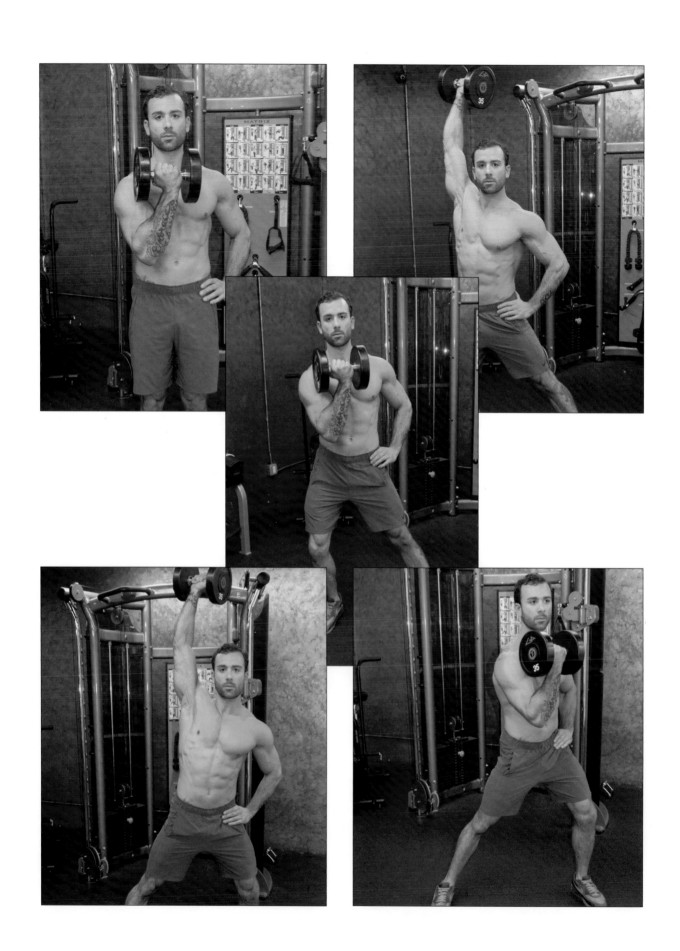

INTRINSIC STRENGTH TRAINING

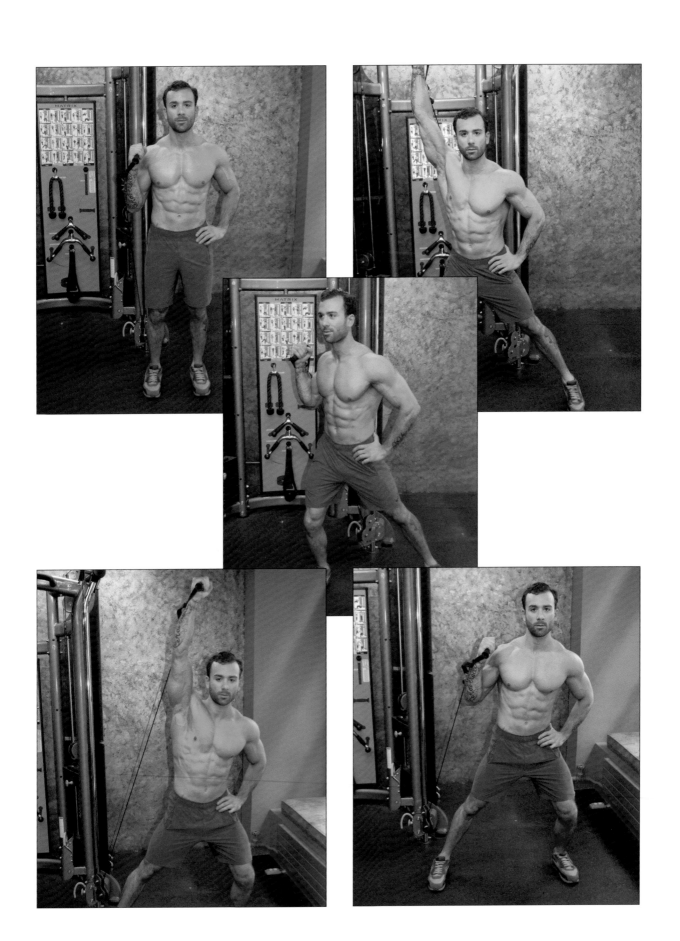

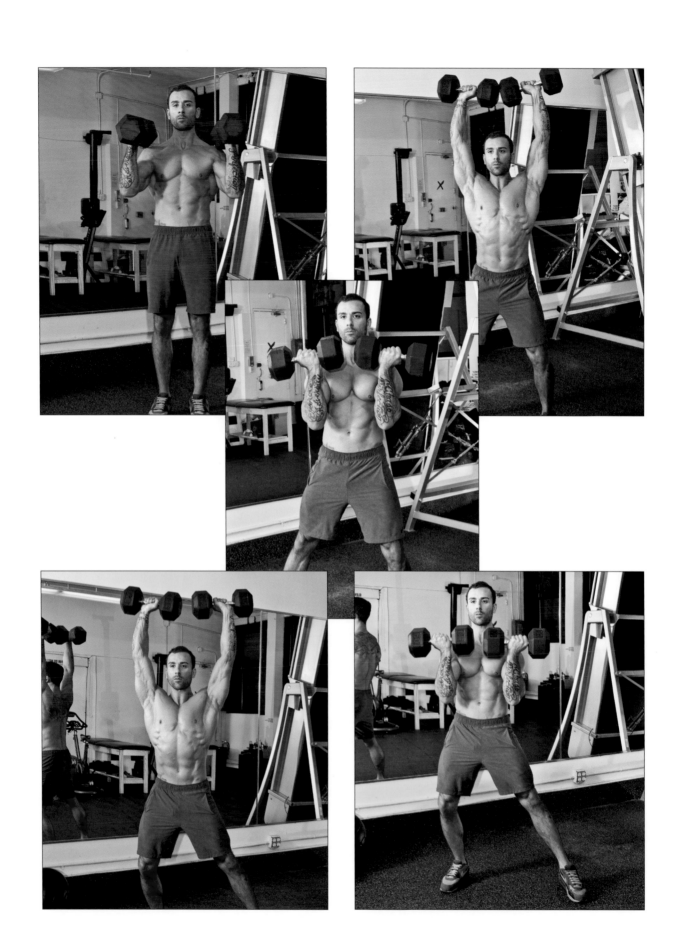

INTRINSIC STRENGTH TRAINING

REPLACEMENT EXERCISE FOR SHOULDER/MILITARY PRESS
IST: OPEN BODY OVERHEAD PRESS

BOS - bilateral start position - back facing - rear rotation step
   (same side foot as resistance)
POR - pelvis height cable - one arm shoulder press overhead

1. Set up with a bilateral stance while back facing the resistance point set at hip height.
2. Hold one resistance handle at the shoulder with one hand.
3. Perform all three phases of IST with each rep: dynamic acceleration, global repetition, and dynamic deceleration.
4. (Dynamic Acceleration) Take a rear rotation step with the same side as resistance handle—towards the the resistance (BOS)—while simultaneously pressing the cable directly above and behind the shoulder (POR).
5. (Global Repetition) Remain in this stance (one foot rear rotated) and execute one complete rotational press by bringing the handle back to the shoulder and pressing back up overhead. (POR)
6. (Dynamic Deceleration) Return to the bilateral starting position (BOS) while bringing the resistance (POR) back to at the shoulder.
7. Repeat for the number of repetitions required by your program.

ANGELO'S ADVICE

1. Focus on using your entire body for this exercise.
2. Allow the ankles, knees, hips, and shoulders to move as needed for full body muscle activation—but with precise control during each part of the exercise.
3. Actively press the forefoot and big toe of the non stepping leg into the ground—activating and stabilizing the entire core to maintain body control, balance, and alignment.
4. Feel free to move pivot the non stepping leg as needed
5. Start with your head in a forward-facing, neutral position.
6. Allow your eyes to follow the resistance handle as you press to ensure core rotation.
7. Focus on using the musculature of the scapula.

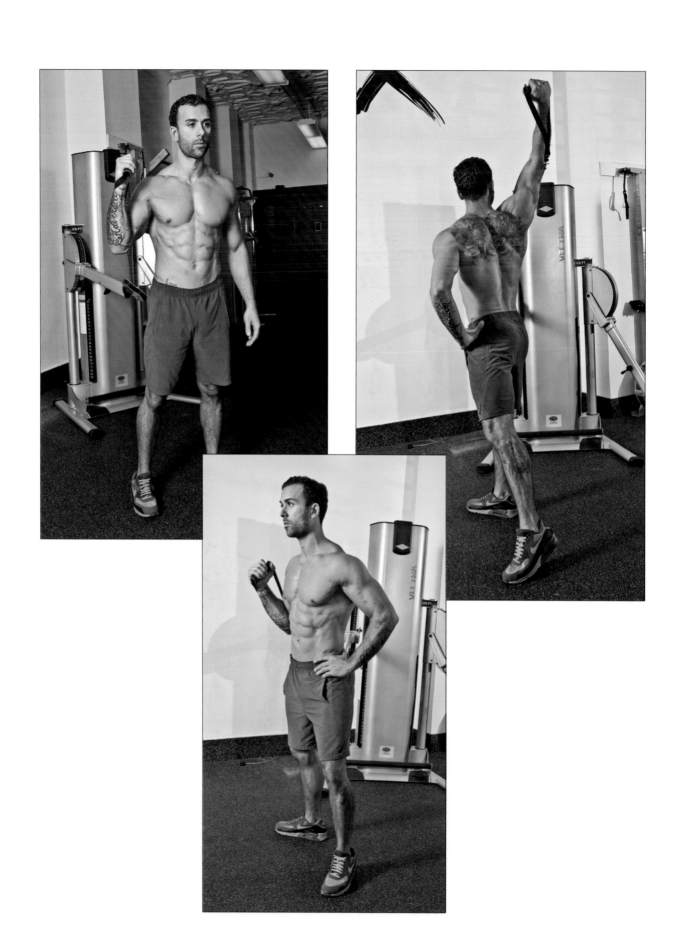

INTRINSIC STRENGTH TRAINING

REPLACEMENT EXERCISE FOR SHOULDER/MILITARY PRESS
IST: REAR ROTATIONAL STEP ROTATING PRESS

BOS - bilateral start position - rear rotation step (same side as the resistance point)
POR - dumbbell, kettlebell - shoulder height - rotate body with shoulder rotation press

1. Set up with a bilateral stance while holding a hand weight at shoulder height with one hand.
2. Perform all three phases of IST with each rep: dynamic acceleration, global repetition, and dynamic deceleration.
3. (Dynamic Acceleration) Take a rear rotation step away from the start position (BOS)—while simultaneously pressing the arm upward above and behind the shoulder (POR).
4. Pivot the non stepping leg towards the end range of body rotation and press.
5. (Global Repetition) Remain in this stance (rear rotation step) and execute one complete shoulder press by pulling the arm back to the sternum at shoulder height and extend directly above and behind the shoulder (POR).
6. (Dynamic Deceleration) Return back to the bilateral starting position (BOS) while bringing the resistance (POR) back to shoulder height.
7. Repeat for the number of repetitions required by your program.

ANGELO'S ADVICE

1. Focus on using your entire body for this exercise.
2. Allow the ankles, knees, hips, and shoulders to move as needed for full body muscle activation —but with precise control during each part of the exercise.
3. Actvely press the forefoot and big toe of the non-stepping leg into the ground—activating and stabilizing the entire core to maintain body control, balance, and alignment.
4. Focus on consistent core tension as you pivot the non-stepping foot.
5. Allow your eyes to follow the resistance handle as you press to ensure core rotation.
6. Focus on using the musculature of the scapula.

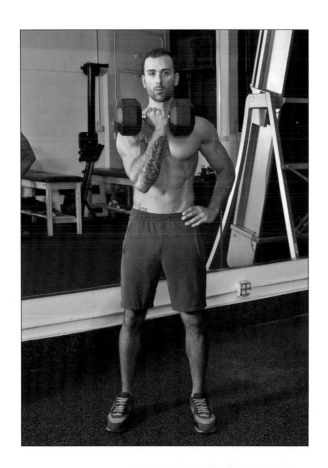
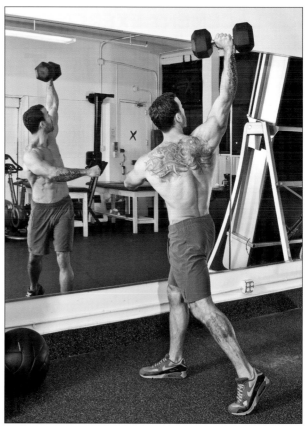
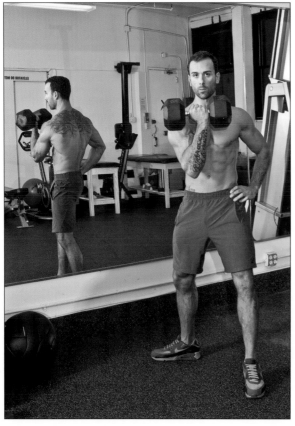
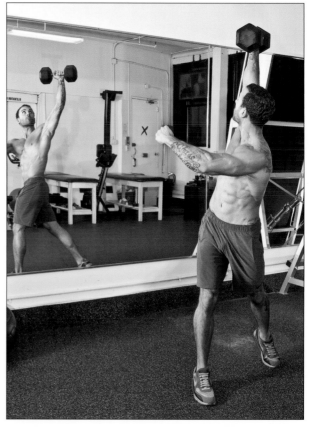

INTRINSIC STRENGTH TRAINING

REPLACEMENT EXERCISE FOR
DELTOID RAISES AND EXTENSIONS
IST: SIDE STEP WITH LATERAL DELTOID RAISE

BOS - bilateral start position - rear rotation step (same side as the resistance point)
POR - dumbbell, kettlebell - shoulder height - rotate body with shoulder rotation press

1.   Set up with a bilateral stance while holding a hand weight at pelvis height with one hand.
2.   Perform all three phases of IST with each rep: dynamic acceleration, global repetition, and dynamic deceleration.
3.   (Dynamic Acceleration) Take a side step away from the start position (BOS)— while simultaneously raising the arm directly to the side and upward above the shoulder (POR).
4.   (Global Repetition) Remain in this stance (side step) and execute one complete shoulder raise by allowing the hand weight to come back to the midline of the body at pelvis height before raising back to shoulder height (POR).
5.   (Dynamic Deceleration) Return back to the bilateral starting position (BOS) while bringing the resistance (POR) back to pelvis height
6.   Repeat for the number of repetitions required by your program.

ANGELO'S ADVICE

1.   Focus on using your entire body for this exercise.
2.   Allow the ankles, knees, hips, and shoulders to move as needed for full body muscle activation—but with precise control during each part of the exercise.
3.   Actively press the forefoot and big toe of the non stepping leg into the ground—activating and stabilizing the entire core to maintain body control, balance, and alignment.
4.   Keep the thumb towards the sky!
5.   Keep your head in a forward-facing, neutral position.

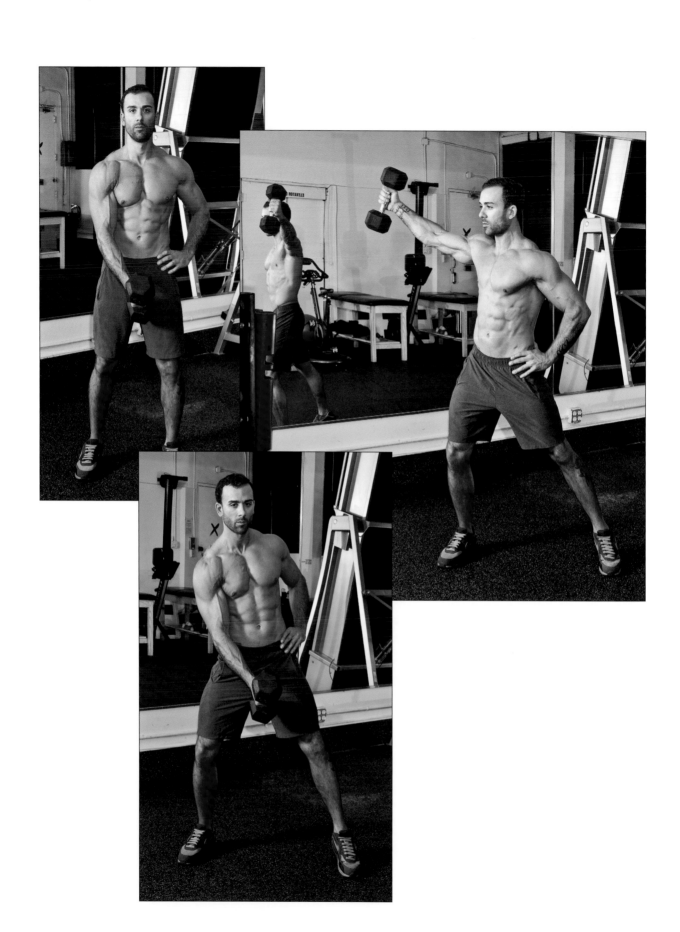

REPLACEMENT EXERCISE FOR DELTOID RAISES AND EXTENSIONS
IST: FORWARD STEP FRONT RAISE

BOS - bilateral start position - back facing - alternating forward step
POR - pelvis height - hand weight - forward raise above shoulder

1. Set up with a bilateral stance while holding a hand weight at pelvis height with one hand.
2. Perform all three phases of IST with each rep: dynamic acceleration, global repetition, and dynamic deceleration.
3. (Dynamic Acceleration) Take a forward step away from the start position (BOS)—while simultaneously raising the arm directly in front and upward above the shoulder. (POR).
4. (Global Repetition) Remain in this stance (forward step) and execute one complete shoulder raise by allowing the hand weight to come back to the pelvis height before raising back up to shoulder height (POR).
5. (Dynamic Deceleration) Return back to the bilateral starting position (BOS) while bringing the resistance (POR) back to pelvis height.
6. Repeat by stepping forward with the opposite foot.

ANGELO'S ADVICE

1. Focus on using your entire body for this exercise.
2. Allow the ankles, knees, hips, and shoulders to move as needed for full body muscle activation—but with precise control during each part of the exercise.
3. Actively press the forefoot and big toe of the non stepping leg into the ground—activating and stabilizing the entire core to maintain body control, balance, and alignment.
4. Keep the thumb towards the sky!
5. Keep your head in a forward-facing, neutral position.

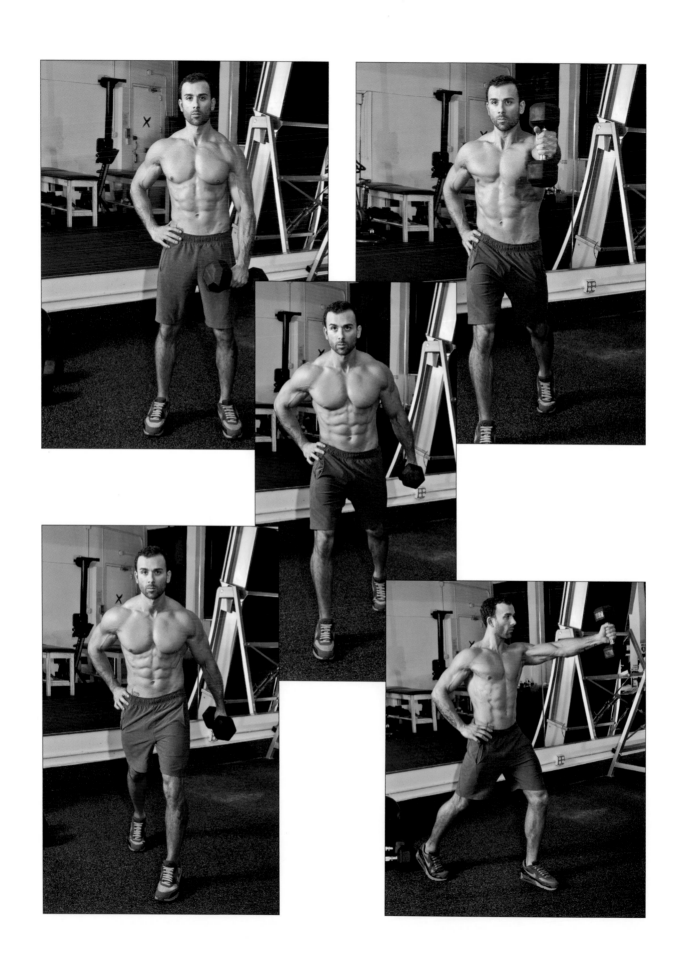

CABLE VARIATION WITH ALTERNATING REAR STEP

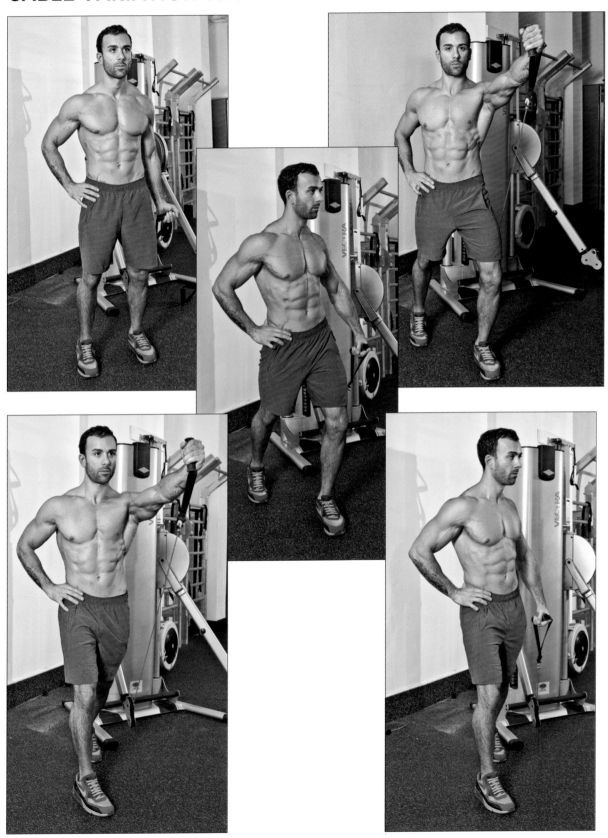

REPLACEMENT EXERCISE FOR
DELTOID RAISES AND EXTENSIONS
IST: REAR ROTATIONAL STEP SHOULDER RAISE

BOS - bilateral start position - rear rotation step (same side as resistance)
POR - dumbbell - shoulder height - one arm rear shoulder lateral extension (fly)

1. Set up with a bilateral stance while holding a hand weight at pelvis height with one hand.
2. Perform all three phases of IST with each rep: dynamic acceleration, global repetition, and dynamic deceleration.
3. (Dynamic Acceleration) Take a rear rotation step away from the start position with the same side foot as the weighted arm (BOS)—while simultaneously raising the arm above the shoulder. (POR).
4. (Global Repetition) Remain in this stance (rear rotation step) and execute one complete shoulder raise by allowing the hand weight to come back to the bodies mid line before raising back up to shoulder height. (POR).
5. (Dynamic Deceleration) Return back to the bilateral starting position (BOS) while bringing the resistance (POR) back to pelvis height.
6. Repeat for the number of repetitions required by your program.

ANGELO'S ADVICE

1. Focus on using your entire body for this exercise.
2. Allow the ankles, knees, hips, and shoulders to move as needed for full body muscle activation—but with precise control during each part of the exercise.
3. Actively press the forefoot and big toe of the non stepping leg into the ground—activating and stabilizing the entire core to maintain body control, balance, and alignment.
4. Keep the thumb towards the sky!
5. Keep your head in a forward-facing, neutral position.

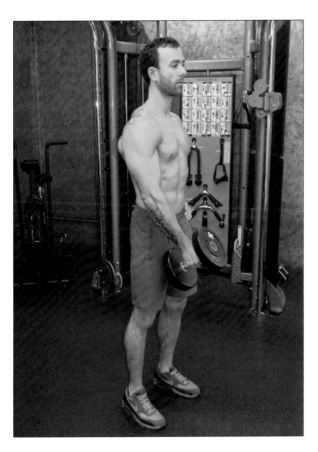

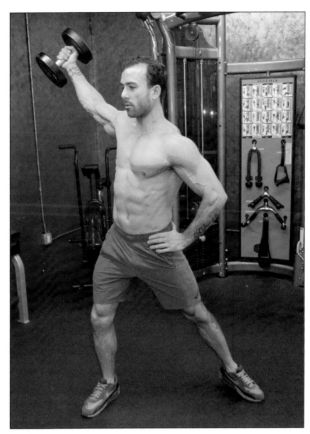

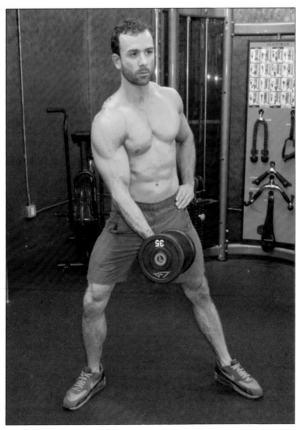

REPLACEMENT EXERCISE FOR
DELTOID RAISES AND EXTENSIONS
IST: FORWARD STEP SHOULDER ACTIVATOR

BOS - bilateral start position - side facing - forward step
POR - ankle height - PNF - Shoulder extension across body

1. Set up with a bilateral stance while side facing the resistance point set at ankle height.
2. Hold one resistance handle at the shoulder with the hand furthest from the resistance point.
3. Perform all three phases of IST with each rep: dynamic acceleration, global repetition, and dynamic deceleration.
4. (Dynamic Acceleration) Take a forward step with the leg furthest from the resistance point (BOS)—while simultaneously extending the same side arm out to the side and above the shoulder (POR).
5. (Global Repetition) Remain in this stance (forward step) and execute one complete shoulder extension by bringing the handle back across the body to the opposite side hip and pressing back up overhead (POR).
6. (Dynamic Deceleration) Return to the bilateral starting position (BOS) while bringing the resistance (POR) back to at the shoulder.
7. Repeat for the number of repetitions required by your program.

ANGELO'S ADVICE

1. Focus on using your entire body for this exercise.
2. Allow the ankles, knees, hips, and shoulders to move as needed for full body muscle activation—but with precise control during each part of the exercise.
3. Actively press the forefoot and big toe of the non stepping leg into the ground—activating and stabilizing the entire core to maintain body control, balance, and alignment.
4. Keep your head in a forward-facing, neutral position.
5. Focus on using the musculature of the scapula.

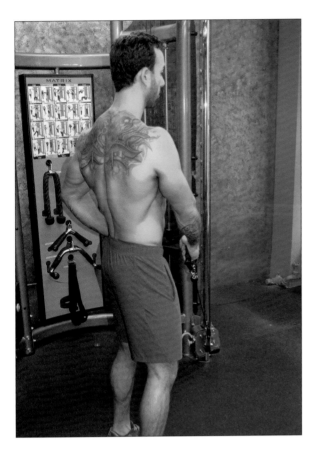

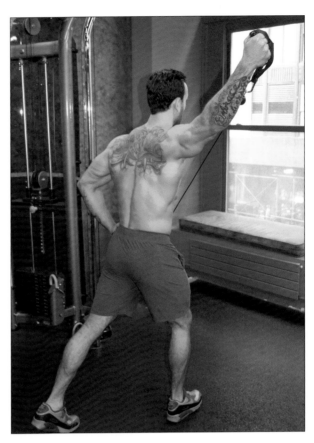

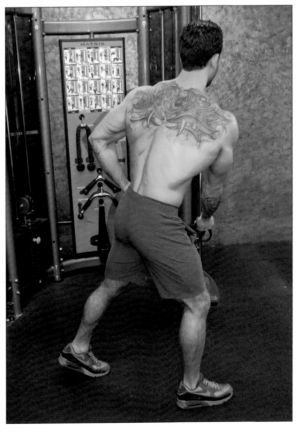

REPLACEMENT EXERCISE FOR
THE STANDARD DIP
IST DIP

BOS - bilateral hand position on dip or parallel bars - supporting body at hip height
POR - dip - global rotation - eyes gaze over and behind the shoulder at bottom of each rep

1. Grip the parallel bars or dip bars with your hands shoulder width apart.
2. Complete a regular dip.
3. Complete a second dip while gazing over the back of the right shoulder at the bottom of the rep.
4. Complete a third dip while gazing over the back of the left shoulder at the bottom of the rep.
5. Perform a series of three dips to complete one repetition of IST dips.
    a. First dip: look over the right shoulder.
    b. Second dip: look straight ahead.
    c. Third dip: look over left shoulder.

ANGELO'S ADVICE

1. Allow every joint to help with the full body rotation.
2. Your eyes will direct your head, shoulders, spine, and hips to rotate towards the same side as focal point (looking behind the shoulder).
3. Actively apply pressure into the bar through your shoulders and fingers to create more tension to radiate through the upper body into the core.

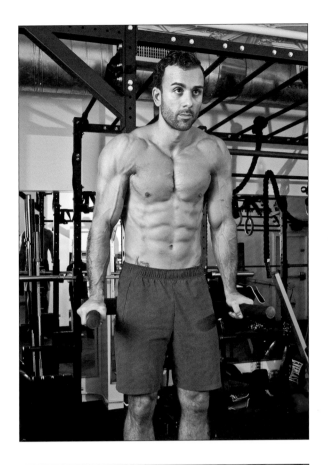
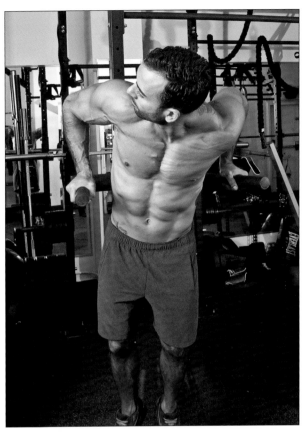
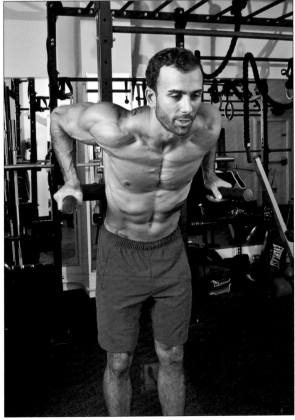
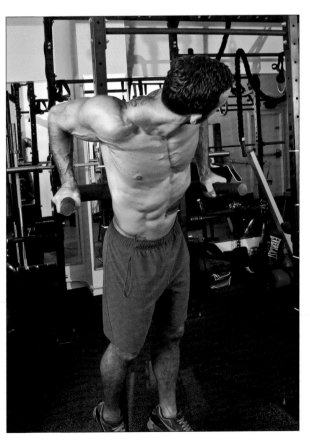

REPLACEMENT EXERCISE FOR UPRIGHT ROW AND HIGH PULL
IST REAR ROTATION STEP HIGH PULL (CABLE EXAMPLE)

BOS - bilateral start position - front facing - rear rotation step
POR - cable - ankle height - row above shoulder

1. Set up with a bilateral stance while facing the resistance point set at ankle height.
2. Hold one resistance handle at the pelvis with the hand closest to the resistance point.
3. Perform all three phases of IST with each rep: dynamic acceleration, global repetition, and dynamic deceleration.
4. (Dynamic Acceleration) Take a rear rotation step with the same side leg holding the resistance handle. (BOS)—while simultaneously rowing the arm up to the height of the shoulder. (POR).
5. (Global Repetition) Remain in this stance (rear rotation step) and execute one complete upright row by bringing the handle back to the midline of the body at pelvis height and rowing back up to the shoulder (POR).
6. (Dynamic Deceleration) Return to the bilateral starting position (BOS) while bringing the resistance (POR) back to at the pelvis.
7. Repeat for the number of repetitions required by your program.

ANGELO'S ADVICE

1. Focus on using your entire body for this exercise.
2. Allow the ankles, knees, hips, and shoulders to move as needed for full body muscle activation—but with precise control during each part of the exercise.
3. Actively press the forefoot and big toe of the non stepping leg into the ground—activating and stabilizing the entire core to maintain body control, balance, and alignment.
4. Feel free to move pivot the non stepping leg as needed.
5. Keep your head in a forward-facing, neutral position.

CABLE EXAMPLE

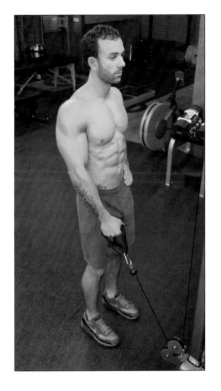 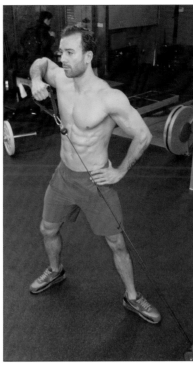 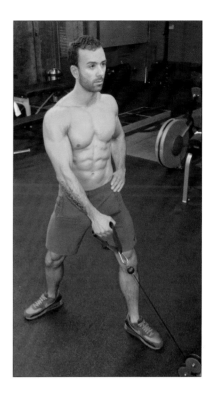

HAND WEIGHT EXAMPLE

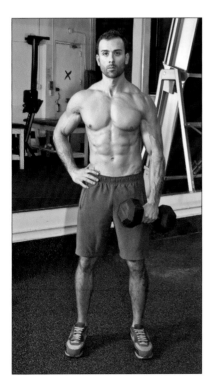 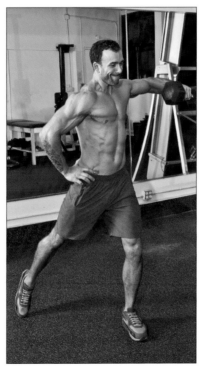 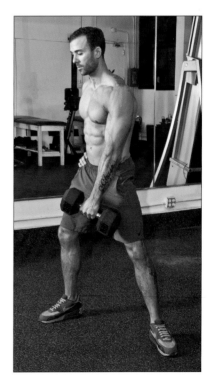

REPLACEMENT EXERCISE FOR
UPRIGHT ROW AND HIGH PULL
IST: FORWARD STEP HIGH PULL (HANDWEIGHT EXAMPLE)

BOS - bilateral start position - alternating forward step
POR - dumbbell, kettlebell, cable - hip height - row to above shoulder

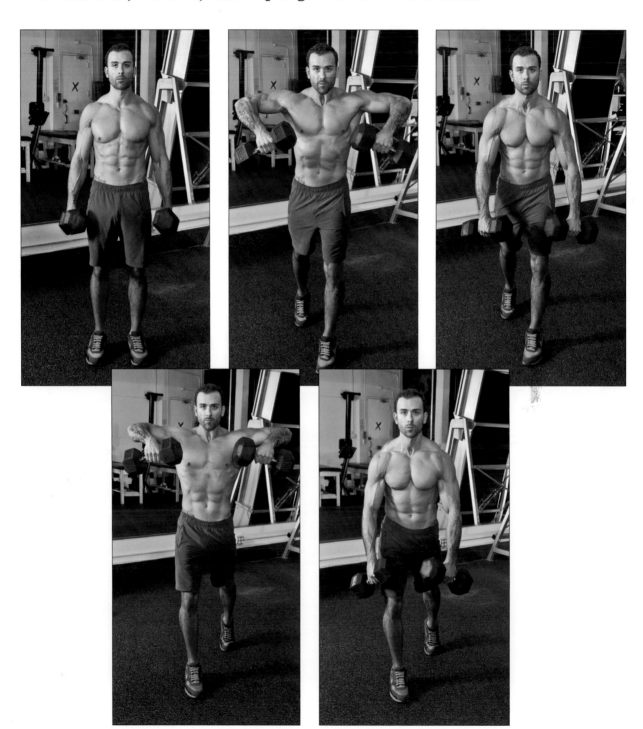

REPLACEMENT EXERCISE FOR
UPRIGHT ROW AND HIGH PULL
IST: SIDE STEP HIGH PULL (HANDWEIGHT EXAMPLE)

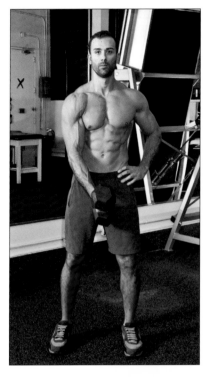

BOS - bilateral start position - side step
    (same side as resistance)
POR - dumbbell, kettlebell, cable - hip height -
    row to above shoulder

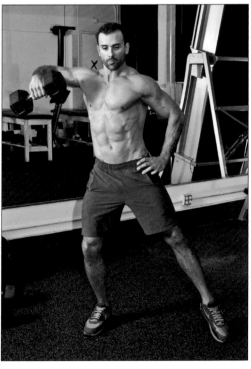

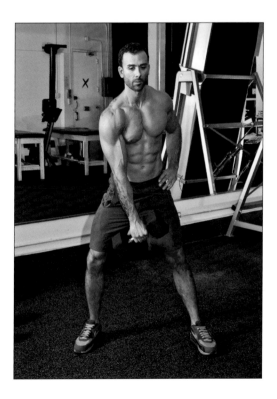

REPLACEMENT EXERCISE FOR
UPRIGHT ROW AND HIGH PULL
IST: REAR STEP HIGH PULL (CABLE EXAMPLE TWO ARM)

BOS - bilateral start position - side facing - alternating rear step
POR - dumbbell, kettlebell, cable - ankle height - row to above shoulder

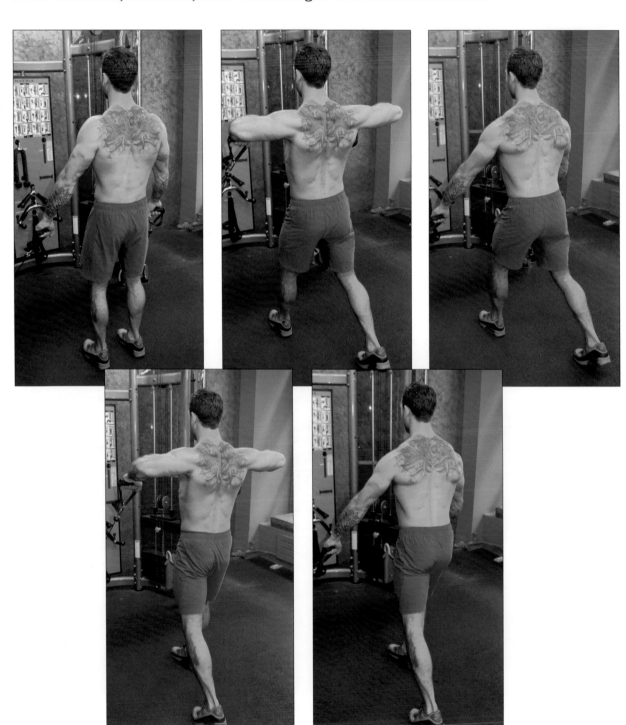

REPLACEMENT EXERCISE FOR
UPRIGHT ROW AND HIGH PULL
IST: REAR STEP HIGH PULL (CABLE EXAMPLE ONE ARM)

BOS - bilateral start position - side facing - alternating rear step
POR - dumbbell, kettlebell, cable - ankle height - row to above shoulder

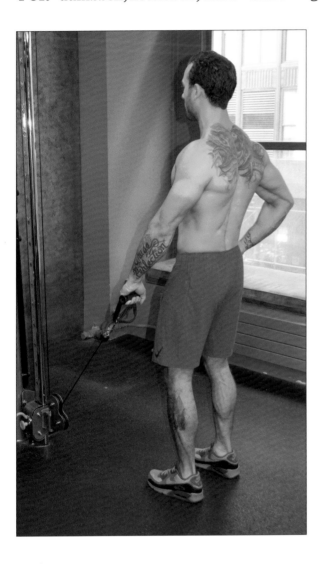
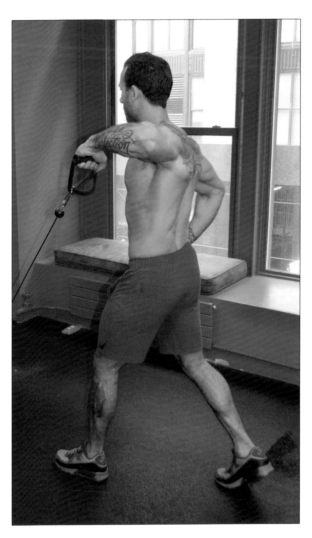

REPLACEMENT EXERCISE FOR
SHOULDER SHRUG
IST REAR STEP SHRUG

BOS - bilateral start position - front facing - alternating rear step
POR - cable - ankle height - shrug shoulders

1. Set up with a bilateral stance while facing the resistance point set at ankle height.
2. Hold both resistance handles at the pelvis
3. Perform all three phases of IST with each rep: dynamic acceleration, global repetition, and dynamic deceleration.
4. (Dynamic Acceleration) Take a rear step with one leg (BOS)— while simultaneously shrugging both arms up at the height of the shoulder (POR).
5. (Global Repetition) Remain in this stance (rear step) and execute one complete shoulder shrug by lowering the shoulders and squeezing them upward again (POR).
6. (Dynamic Deceleration) Return to the bilateral starting position (BOS) while bringing the shoulders back to their starting position.
7. Repeat by stepping the opposite foot backwards.

ANGELO'S ADVICE

1. Focus on using your entire body for this exercise.
2. Allow the ankles, knees, hips, and shoulders to move as needed for full body muscle activation—but with precise control during each part of the exercise.
3. Actively press the forefoot and big toe of both legs into the ground—activating and stabilizing the entire core to maintain body control, balance, and alignment.
4. Keep your head in a forward-facing, neutral position.

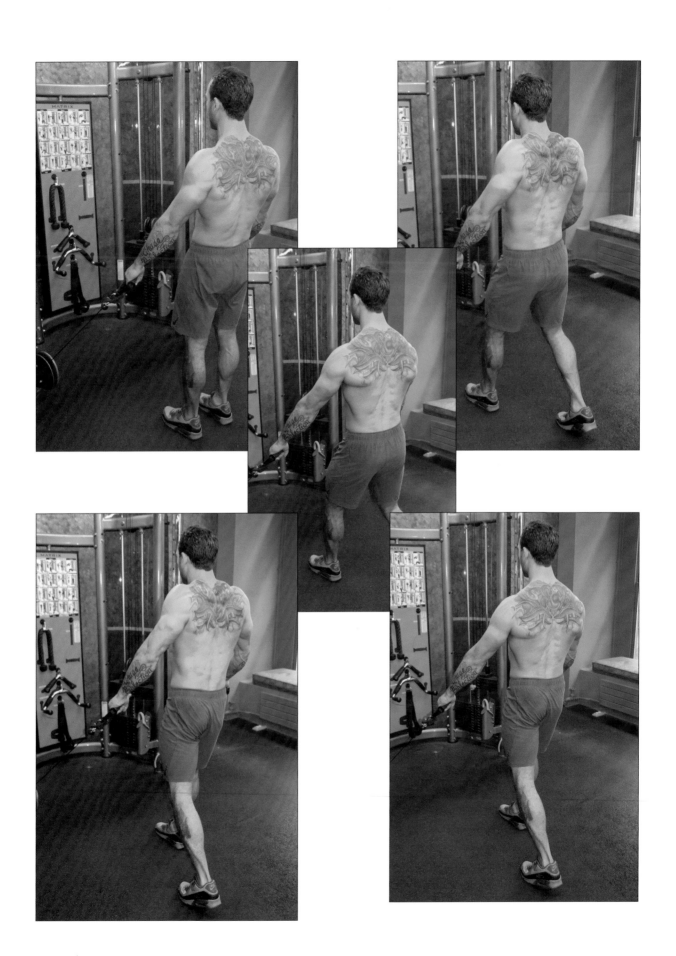

REPLACEMENT EXERCISE FOR
UPRIGHT ROW AND HIGH PULL
IST: FORWARD STEP SHRUG

BOS - bilateral start position - front facing - alternating forward step
POR - cable - ankle height - shrug shoulders

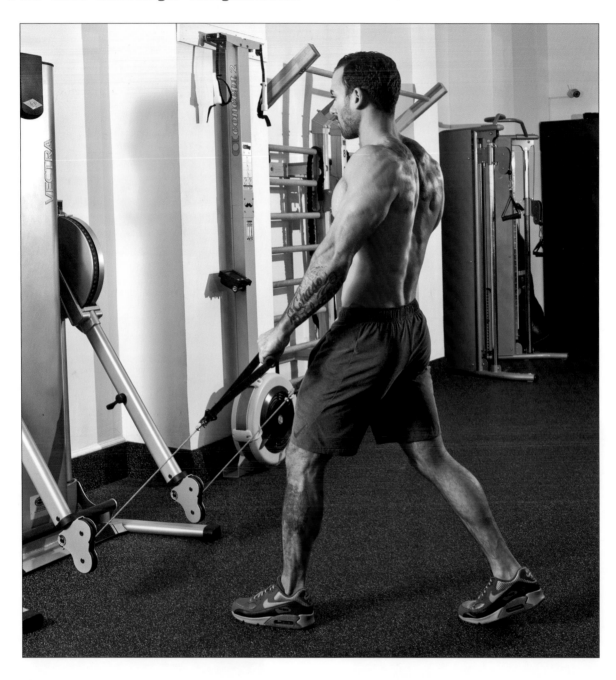

INTRINSIC STRENGTH TRAINING

REPLACEMENT EXERCISE FOR
UPRIGHT ROW AND HIGH PULL
IST: SIDE STEP SHRUG (BARBELL EXAMPLE)

BOS - bilateral start position - side step
POR – barbell - hip height - shrug shoulders

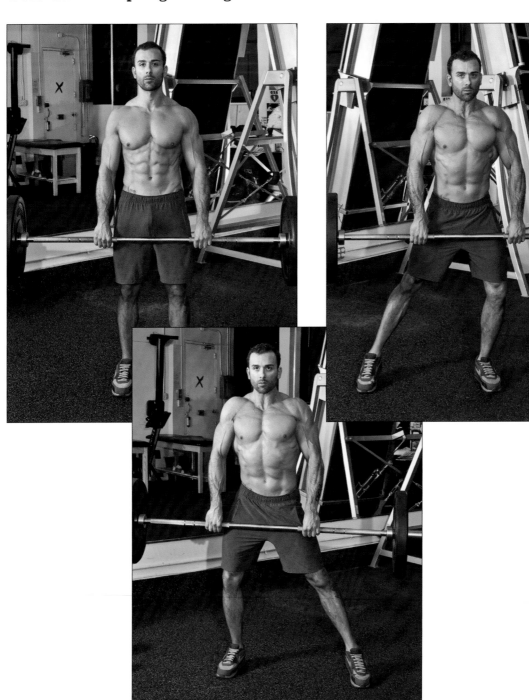

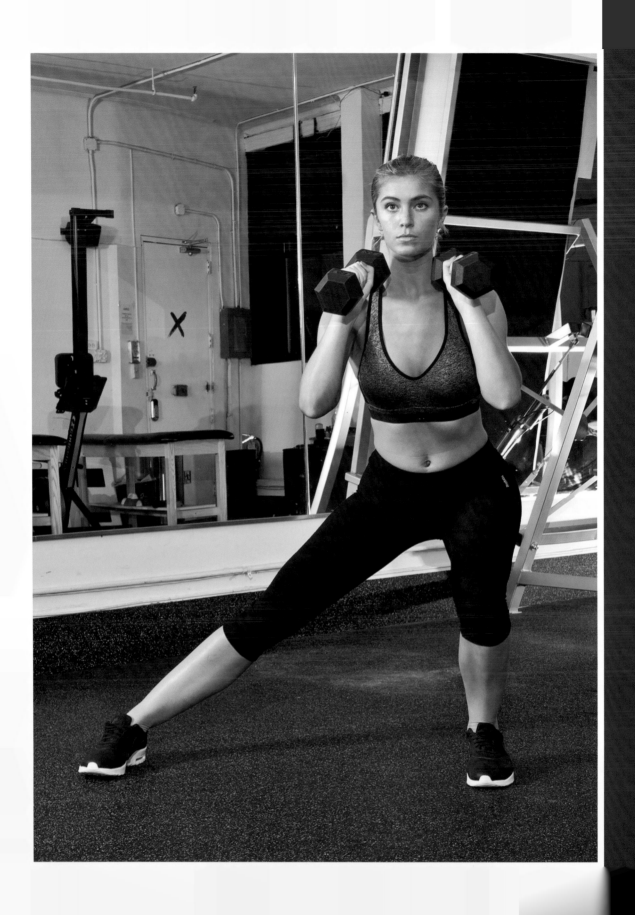

Limitless Legs

W e carry, push, and pull things every day with our arms. But without using our legs, those objects aren't going anywhere. When we carry, push, or pull a given item, how often are we standing with our feet perfectly even and shoulder width apart? Are we trying to do these tasks while sitting down or while taking huge dramatic lunges? The answer is no, instead our feet are usually taking small steps. Think about the last time you carried or pushed something large and heavy from point A to point B. Did you take massive lunges to get there, or were you using small, controlled steps?

We initiate all of our movements by stepping, so let's start approaching exercise with efficient steps.

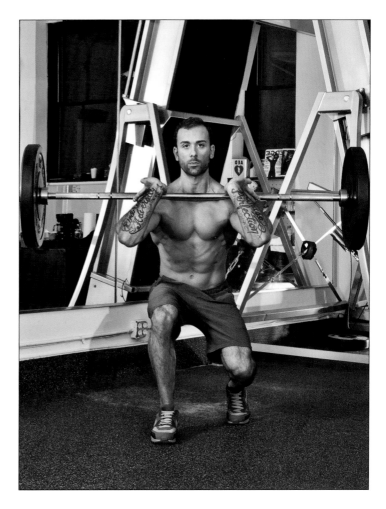

REPLACEMENT EXERCISE FOR DEADLIFTS
IST: FORWARD STEP DEADLIFT

BOS - bilateral start position - alternating forward step
POR - hand weight - hip height- deadlift

1.   Set up with a bilateral stance while holding a hand weight at pelvis height with both hands.
2.   Perform all three phases of IST with each rep: dynamic acceleration, global repetition, and dynamic deceleration.
3.   (Dynamic Acceleration) Take a forward step away from the start position (BOS)—while simultaneously lowering the weight towards the floor. (POR).
4.   (Global Repetition) Remain in this stance (forward step) and execute one complete deadlift by raising the weight back to the height of the hip and standing upright. Lower the weight back to the floor by hinging the hips (POR).
5.   (Dynamic Deceleration) Return back to the bilateral starting position (BOS) while bringing the hand weight (POR) back to pelvis height
6.   Repeat by stepping forward with the opposite foot.
7.   Variations to Deadlifts—use one or both hands are holding a weight (barbell, medicine ball, kettlebell, dumbbell, etc.)

ANGELO'S ADVICE

1.   Focus on using your entire body for this exercise.
2.   Allow the ankles, knees, hips, and shoulders to move as needed for full body muscle activation—but with precise control during each part of the exercise.
3.   Transfer the bodies weight into the forward stepping leg
4.   Actively press the forefoot and big toe both leg into the ground—activating and stabilizing the entire core to maintain body control, balance, and alignment.
5.   Take your time to allow the glutes, thighs, hamstrings, and core to integrate and control the resistance forces together.

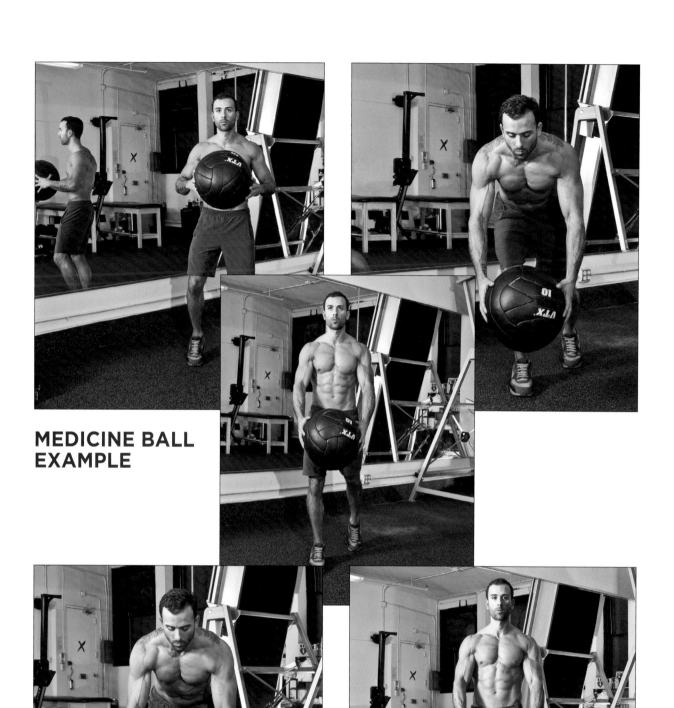

MEDICINE BALL
EXAMPLE

REPLACEMENT EXERCISE FOR DEADLIFTS
IST: REAR STEP DEADLIFT

BOS - bilateral start position - alternating rear step
POR - Hand weight – hip height - deadlift

1.   Set up with a bilateral stance while holding a hand weight at pelvis height with both hands.
2.   Perform all three phases of IST with each rep: dynamic acceleration, global repetition, and dynamic deceleration.
3.   (Dynamic Acceleration) Take a rear step toe reach away from the start position (BOS)— while simultaneously lowering the weight towards the floor. (POR).
4.   (Global Repetition) Remain in this stance (rear step toe reach) and execute one complete deadlift by raising the weight back to the height of the hip and standing upright. Lower the weight back to the floor by hinging the hips (POR).
5.   (Dynamic Deceleration) Return back to the bilateral starting position (BOS) while bringing the hand weight (POR) back to pelvis height.
6.   Repeat by stepping behind with the opposite foot.

ANGELO'S ADVICE

1.   Focus on using your entire body for this exercise.
2.   Allow the ankles, knees, hips, and shoulders to move as needed for full body muscle activation—but with precise control during each part of the exercise.
3.   Leave the majority of the bodies weight on the non stepping leg
4.   Actively press the forefoot and big toe both legs into the groundactivating and stabilizing the entire core to maintain body control, balance, and alignment.
5.   Take your time to allow the glutes, thighs, hamstrings, and core to integrate and control the resistance forces together.
6.   Be sure to keep a strong and erect posture by applying tension throughout the core, keeping the spine and head in a neutral position.

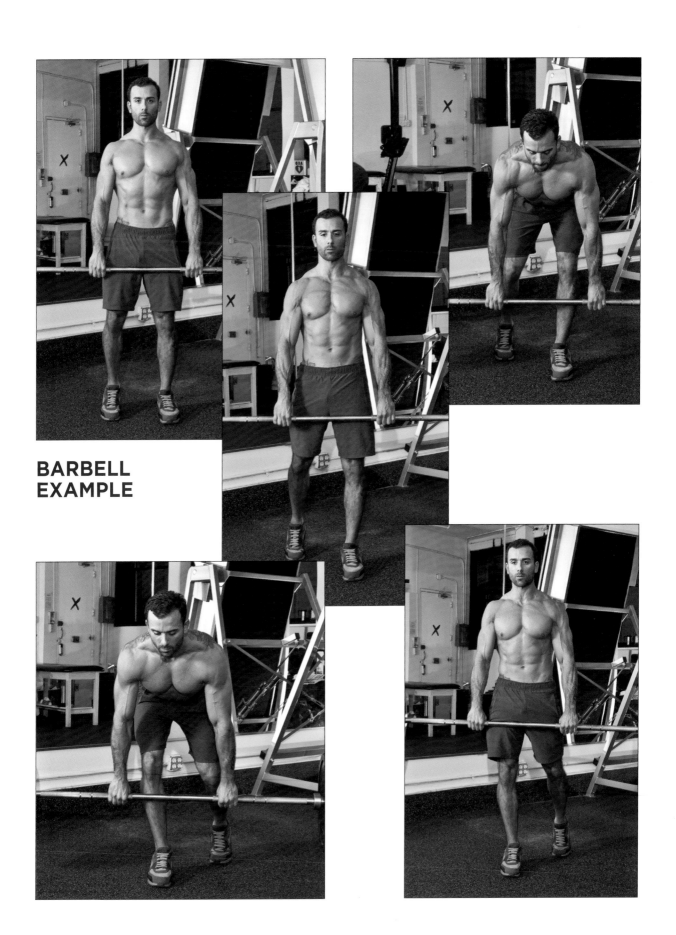

**BARBELL
EXAMPLE**

REPLACEMENT EXERCISE FOR DEADLIFTS
IST: SIDE STEP DEADLIFT

BOS - bilateral start position - alternating side step
POR - Hand weight – hip height - deadlift

1. Set up with a bilateral stance while holding a hand weight at pelvis height with both hands.
2. Perform all three phases of IST with each rep: dynamic acceleration, global repetition, and dynamic deceleration.
3. (Dynamic Acceleration) Take a side step toe reach away from the start position (BOS) while simultaneously lowering the weight towards the floor. (POR).
4. (Global Repetition) Remain in this stance (side step toe reach) and execute one complete deadlift by raising the weight back to the height of the hip and standing upright. Lower the weight back to the floor by hinging the hips. (POR)
5. (Dynamic Deceleration) Return back to the bilateral starting position (BOS) while bringing the hand weight (POR) back to pelvis height.
6. Repeat by stepping the opposite foot to the opposite side.

ANGELO'S ADVICE

1. Focus on using your entire body for this exercise.
2. Allow the ankles, knees, hips, and shoulders to move as needed for full body muscle a ctivation—but with precise control during each part of the exercise.
3. Leave the majority of the bodies weight on the non stepping leg.
4. Actively press the forefoot and big toe both legs into the ground—activating and stabilizing the entire core to maintain body control, balance, and alignment.
5. Take your time to allow the glutes, thighs, hamstrings, and core to integrate and control the resistance forces together.
6. Be sure to keep a strong and erect posture by applying tension throughout the core, keeping the spine and head in a neutral position.

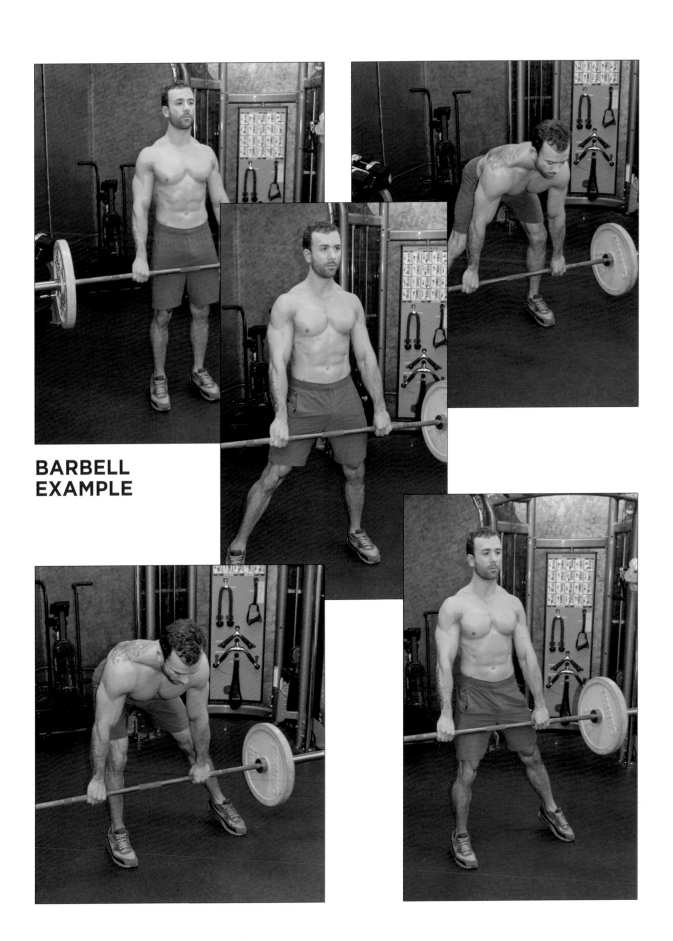

BARBELL EXAMPLE

REPLACEMENT EXERCISE FOR DEADLIFTS
IST: REAR ROTATION STEP DEADLIFT

BOS - bilateral start position - alternating rear rotation step - deadlift
POR - one or both hands hold a barbell, dumbbell, or kettlebell – hip height

1. Set up with a bilateral stance while holding a hand weight at pelvis height with both hands.
2. Perform all three phases of IST with each rep: dynamic acceleration, global repetition, and dynamic deceleration.
3. (Dynamic Acceleration) Take a rear rotation step away from the start position (BOS)—while simultaneously lowering the weight towards the floor. (POR).
4. (Global Repetition) Remain in this stance (rear rotation step) and execute one complete deadlift by raising the weight back to the height of the hip and standing upright. Lower the weight back to the floor by hinging the hips (POR).
5. (Dynamic Deceleration) Return back to the bilateral starting position (BOS) while bringing the hand weight (POR) back to pelvis height.
6. Repeat by stepping the opposite foot to the opposite side.

ANGELO'S ADVICE

1. Focus on using your entire body for this exercise.
2. Allow the ankles, knees, hips, and shoulders to move as needed for full body muscle activation—but with precise control during each part of the exercise.
3. Leave the majority of the bodies weight on the non stepping leg.
4. Actively press the forefoot and big toe both legs into the ground—activating and stabilizing the entire core to maintain body control, balance, and alignment.
5. Take your time to allow the glutes, thighs, hamstrings, and core to integrate and control the resistance forces together.
6. Be sure to keep a strong and erect posture by applying tension throughout the core, keeping the spine and head in a neutral position.

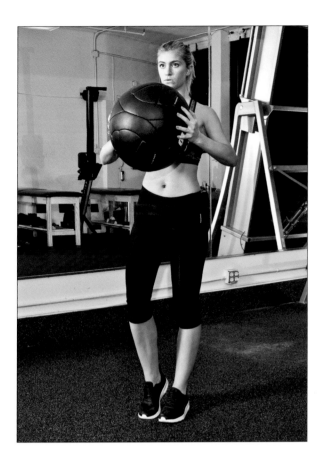

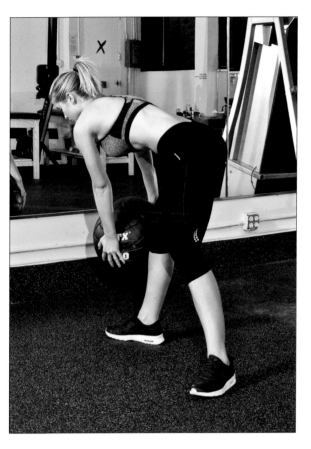

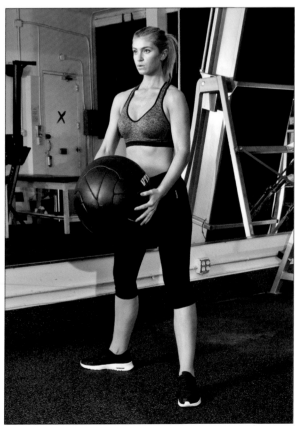

REPLACEMENT EXERCISE FOR
SQUAT PATTERNS AND ALTERNATIVES
IST: FORWARD STEP SQUAT

BOS - bilateral start position - alternating forward step - squat
POR - weight in both hands - front loaded barbell, dumbbells, or kettlebells in rack position

1. Set up with a bilateral stance while holding a hand weight at shoulder height with both hands.
2. Perform all three phases of IST with each rep: dynamic acceleration, global repetition, and dynamic deceleration.
3. (Dynamic Acceleration) -Take a forward step toe reach away from the start position (BOS)— while simultaneously lowering the torso towards the floor (POR).
4. (Global Repetition) - Remain in this stance (forward step toe reach) and execute one complete squat by raising the torso back up to standing height and lowering the torso back down towards the floor (POR).
5. (Dynamic Deceleration) - Return back to the bilateral starting position (BOS) while leaving the hand weights at shoulder height (POR).
6. Repeat by stepping the opposite foot to the opposite side.

ANGELO'S ADVICE

1. Leave the majority of the bodies weight on the non stepping leg.
2. Focus on using your entire body for this exercise.
3. Focus on challenging the butt to sit behind the ankles - keeping the tension in the powerful muscles and out of the knees.
4. Allow the ankles, knees, hips, and shoulders to move as needed for full body muscle activation —but with precise control during each part of the exercise.
5. Actively press the forefoot and big toe both legs into the ground - Activating and stabilizing the entire core to maintain body control, balance, and alignment.
6. Take your time to allow the glutes, thighs, hamstrings, and core to integrate and control the resistance forces together.
7. Be sure to keep a strong and erect posture by applying tension throughout the core, keeping the spine and head in a neutral position.

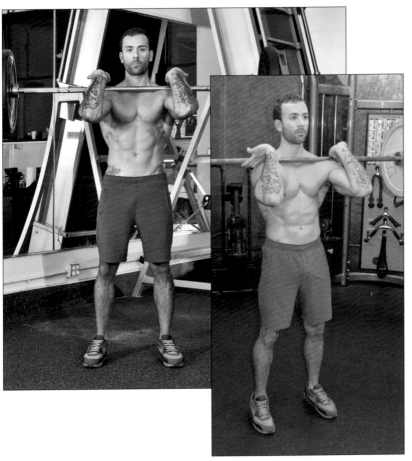
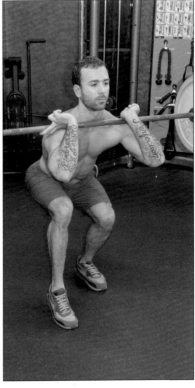
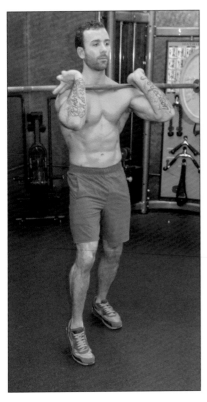
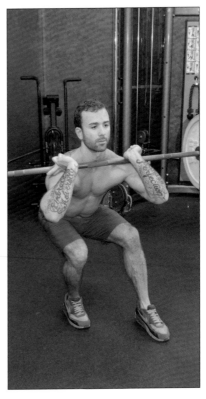
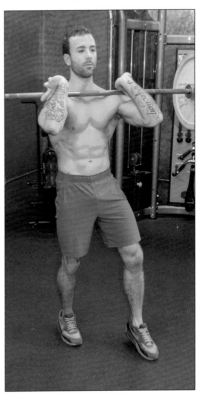

REPLACEMENT EXERCISE FOR
SQUAT PATTERNS AND ALTERNATIVES
IST: REAR STEP SQUAT

BOS - bilateral start position - alternating rear step - squat
POR - weight in both hands - front loaded barbell, dumbbells, or kettlebells in rack position

1. Set up with a bilateral stance while holding a hand weight at shoulder height with both hands.
2. Perform all three phases of IST with each rep: dynamic acceleration, global repetition, and dynamic deceleration.
3. (Dynamic Acceleration) Take a rear step toe reach away from the start position (BOS) while simultaneously lowering the torso towards the floor. (POR).
4. (Global Repetition) Remain in this stance (rear step toe reach) and execute one complete squat by raising the torso back up to standing height and lowering the torso back down towards the floor (POR).
5. (Dynamic Deceleration) Return back to the bilateral starting position (BOS) while leaving the hand weights at shoulder height (POR).
6. Repeat by stepping the opposite foot to the opposite side.

ANGELO'S ADVICE

1. Leave the majority of the bodies weight on the non stepping leg
2. Focus on using your entire body for this exercise.
3. Focus on challenging the butt to sit behind the ankles—keeping the tension in the powerful muscles and out of the knees.
4. Allow the ankles, knees, hips, and shoulders to move as needed for full body muscle activation—but with precise control during each part of the exercise.
5. Actively press the forefoot and big toe both legs into the ground—activating and stabilizing the entire core to maintain body control, balance, and alignment.
6. Take your time to allow the glutes, thighs, hamstrings, and core to integrate and control the resistance forces together.
7. Be sure to keep a strong and erect posture by applying tension throughout the core, keeping the spine and head in a neutral position.

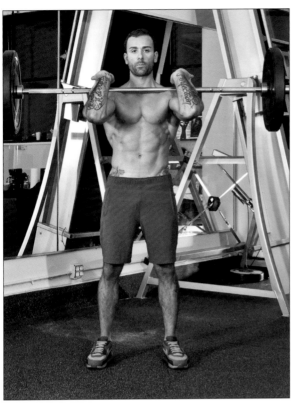
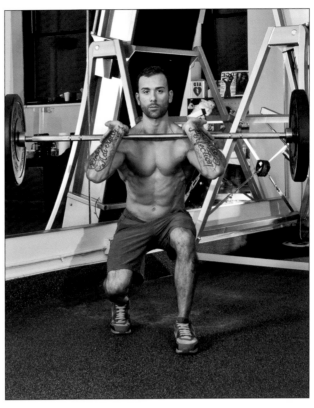
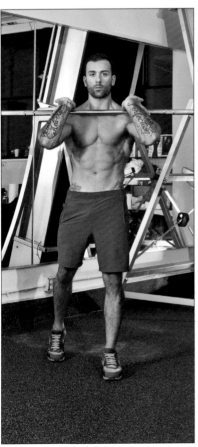
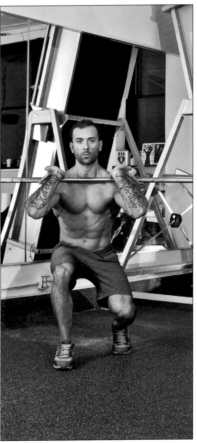
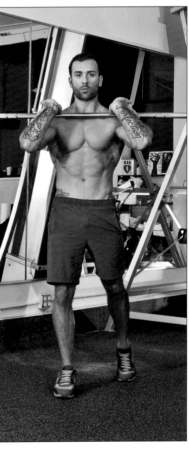

REPLACEMENT EXERCISE FOR
SQUAT PATTERNS AND ALTERNATIVES
IST: SIDE STEP SQUAT

BOS - bilateral start position - alternating side step - squat
POR - weight in both hands - front loaded barbell, dumbbells, or kettlebells
      in rack position

1. Set up with a bilateral stance while holding a hand weight at shoulder height with both hands.
2. Perform all three phases of IST with each rep: dynamic acceleration, global repetition, and dynamic deceleration.
3. (Dynamic Acceleration) Take a side step toe reach away from the start position (BOS) while simultaneously lowering the torso towards the floor. (POR).
4. (Global Repetition) Remain in this stance (side step toe reach) and execute one complete squat by raising the torso back up to standing height and lowering the torso back down towards the floor (POR).
5. (Dynamic Deceleration) Return back to the bilateral starting position (BOS) while leaving the hand weights at shoulder height (POR).
6. Repeat by stepping the opposite foot to the opposite side.

ANGELO'S ADVICE

1. Leave the majority of the bodies weight on the non stepping leg
2. Focus on using your entire body for this exercise.
3. Focus on challenging the butt to sit behind the ankles - keeping the tension in the powerful muscles and out of the knees.
4. Allow the ankles, knees, hips, and shoulders to move as needed for full body muscle activation—but with precise control during each part of the exercise.
5. Actively press the forefoot and big toe both legs into the ground—activating and stabilizing the entire core to maintain body control, balance, and alignment.
6. Take your time to allow the glutes, thighs, hamstrings, and core to integrate and control the resistance forces together.
7. Be sure to keep a strong and erect posture by applying tension throughout the core, keeping the spine and head in a neutral position.

Another variation is to transfer the majority of the body's weight into the stepping leg which will challenge the muscles of the stepping leg much differently compared to the toe reach version.

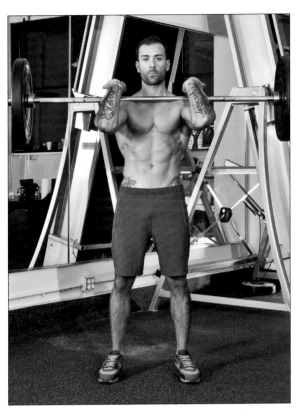

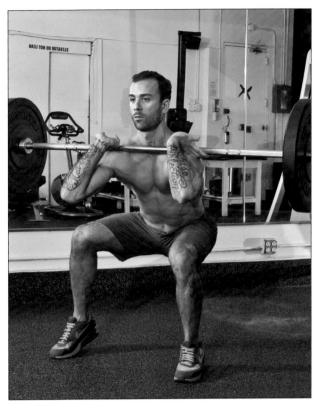

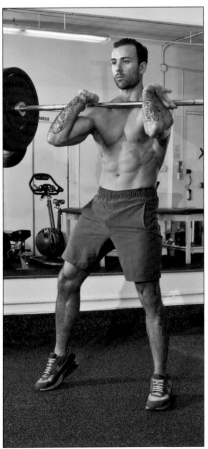

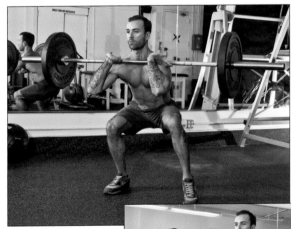

REPLACEMENT EXERCISE FOR
SQUAT PATTERNS AND ALTERNATIVES
IST: REAR ROTATION STEP SQUAT

BOS - bilateral start position - alternating rear rotation step - squat
POR - weight in both hands - front loaded barbell, dumbbells, or kettlebells
   in rack position

1. Set up with a bilateral stance while holding a hand weight at shoulder height with both hands.
2. Perform all three phases of IST with each rep: dynamic acceleration, global repetition, and dynamic deceleration.
3. (Dynamic Acceleration) Take a rear rotation step toe reach away from the start position (BOS)— while simultaneously lowering the torso towards the floor (POR).
4. (Global Repetition) Remain in this stance (rear rotation step toe reach) and execute one complete squat by raising the torso back up to standing height and lowering the torso back down towards the floor (POR).
5. (Dynamic Deceleration) Return back to the bilateral starting position (BOS) while leaving the hand weights at shoulder height (POR).
6. Repeat by stepping the opposite foot to the opposite side.

ANGELO'S ADVICE

1. Leave the majority of the bodies weight on the non stepping leg.
2. Focus on using your entire body for this exercise.
3. Focus on challenging the butt to sit behind the ankles—keeping the tension in the powerful muscles and out of the knees.
4. Allow the ankles, knees, hips, and shoulders to move as needed for full body muscle activation—but with precise control during each part of the exercise.
5. Actvely press the forefoot and big toe both legs into the ground—activating and stabilizing the entire core to maintain body control, balance, and alignment.
6. Take your time to allow the glutes, thighs, hamstrings, and core to integrate and control the resistance forces together.
7. Be sure to keep a strong and erect posture by applying tension throughout the core, keeping the spine and head in a neutral position.

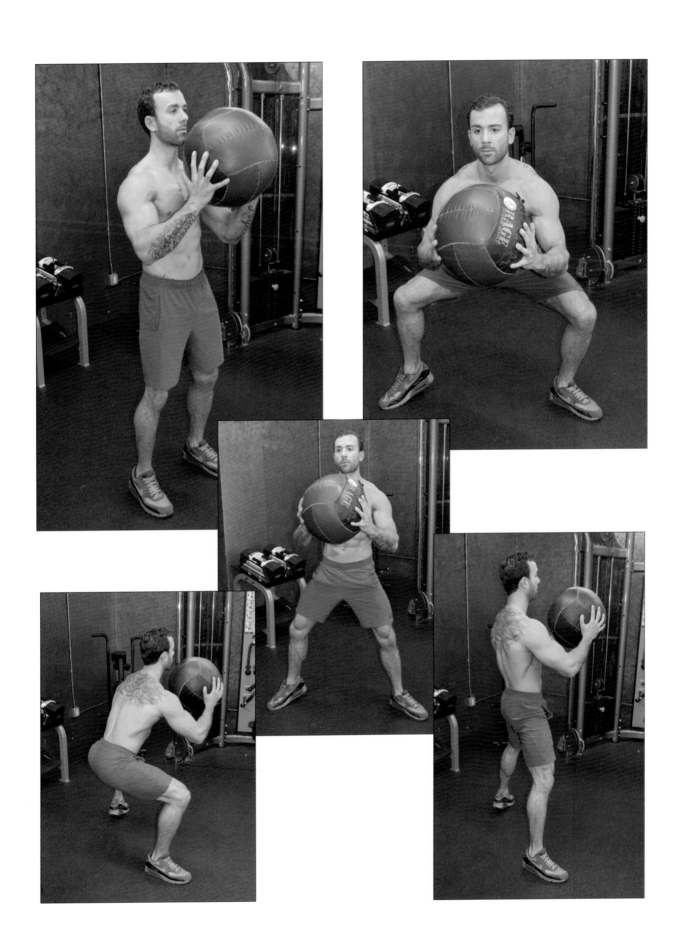

REPLACEMENT EXERCISE FOR
SQUAT PATTERNS AND ALTERNATIVES
IST: REAR ROTATION STEP SQUAT

BOS - bilateral start position - alternating rear rotation step - squat
POR - weight in both hands - front loaded barbell, dumbbells, or kettlebells in rack position

Another variation is to transfer the majority of the body's weight into the stepping leg which will challenge the muscles of the stepping leg much differently compared to the toe reach version.

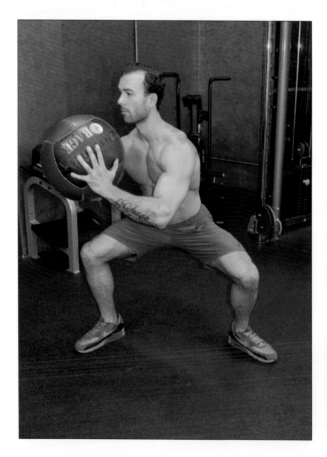
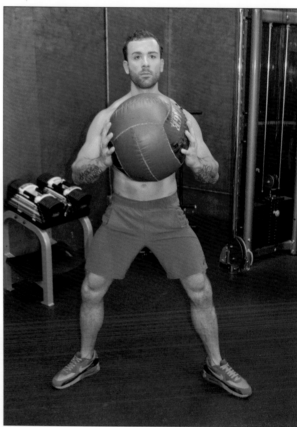

REPLACEMENT EXERCISE FOR
SQUAT PATTERNS AND ALTERNATIVES
IST: ALTERNATING REAR CROSSOVER SQUAT

BOS - bilateral starting position - alternating rear crossover squat
POR - weight in both hands - front loaded barbell, dumbbells, or kettlebells in
rack position

1. Set up with a bilateral stance while holding a hand weight at shoulder height with both hands.
2. Perform all three phases of IST with each rep: dynamic acceleration, global repetition, and dynamic deceleration.
3. (Dynamic Acceleration) - Take a rear cross over step toe reach away from the start position (BOS)— while simultaneously lowering the torso towards the floor. (POR).
4. (Global Repetition) - Remain in this stance (rear cross over step toe reach) and execute one complete squat by raising the torso back up to standing height and lowering the torso back down towards the floor. (POR)
5. (Dynamic Deceleration) - Return back to the bilateral starting position (BOS) while leaving the hand weights at shoulder height (POR)
6. Repeat by stepping the opposite foot to the opposite side.

ANGELO'S ADVICE

1. Leave the majority of the bodies weight on the non stepping leg
2. Focus on using your entire body for this exercise.
3. Focus on challenging the butt to sit behind the ankles - keeping the tension in the powerful muscles and out of the knees.
4. Allow the ankles, knees, hips, and shoulders to move as needed for full body muscle activation —but with precise control during each part of the exercise.
5. Actively press the forefoot and big toe both legs into the ground - Activating and stabilizing the entire core to maintain body control, balance, and alignment.
6. Take your time to allow the glutes, thighs, hamstrings, and core to integrate and control the resistance forces together.
7. Be sure to keep a strong and erect posture by applying tension throughout the core, keeping the spine and head in an neutral position.

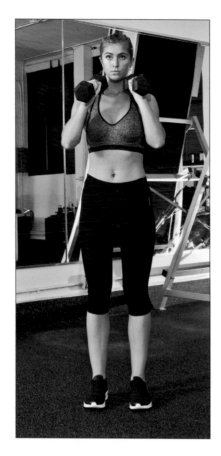
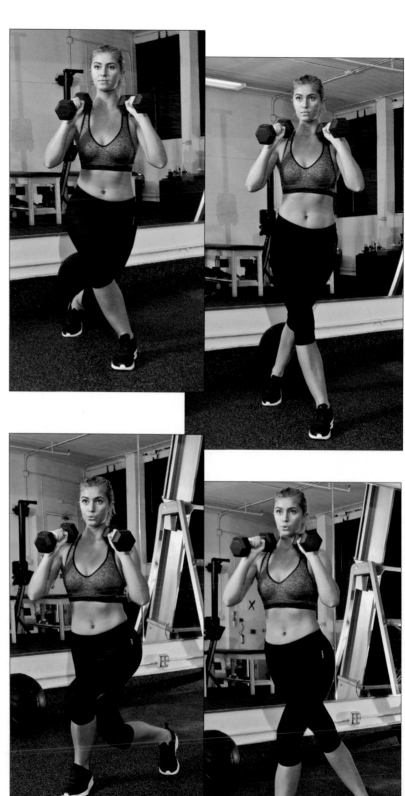

INTRINSIC STRENGTH TRAINING

REPLACEMENT EXERCISE FOR ADDUCTOR/ABDUCTOR MACHINE
IST: ALTERNATING SIDE SQUAT SLIDE

BOS - bilateral start position - side step with single leg squat
POR - one or two hands holding weight at chest height or rack position

Switch sides through half of the set or on every other set.

1. Set up with a bilateral stance while holding a hand weight at shoulder height with both hands.
2. Perform all three phases of IST with each rep: dynamic acceleration, global repetition, and dynamic deceleration.
3. (Dynamic Acceleration) - Take a side step away from the start position (BOS)— while simultaneously lowering the torso towards the floor. (POR).
4. (Global Repetition) - Remain in this stance (side step) and execute one complete squat by raising the torso back up to standing height and lowering the torso back down towards the floor. (POR)
5. (Dynamic Deceleration) - Return back to the bilateral starting position (BOS) while leaving the hand weights at shoulder height (POR)
6. Repeat by stepping the opposite foot to the opposite side.

ANGELO'S ADVICE

1. Load the majority of the bodies weight into the stepping leg.
2. This is necessary to lift up and stabilize the torso as you slide the opposite leg back into a bilateral starting position.
3. Focus on challenging the butt to sit behind the ankles - keeping the tension in the powerful muscles and out of the knees.
4. Focus on using your entire body for this exercise.
5. Allow the ankles, knees, hips, and shoulders to move as needed for full body muscle activation —but with precise control during each part of the exercise.
6. Actively press the forefoot and big toe of the stepping leg into the ground - Activating and stabilizing the entire core to maintain body control, balance, and alignment.
7. Take your time to allow the glutes, thighs, hamstrings, and core to integrate and control the resistance forces together.
8. Be sure to keep a strong and erect posture by applying tension throughout the core, keeping the spine and head in an neutral position.

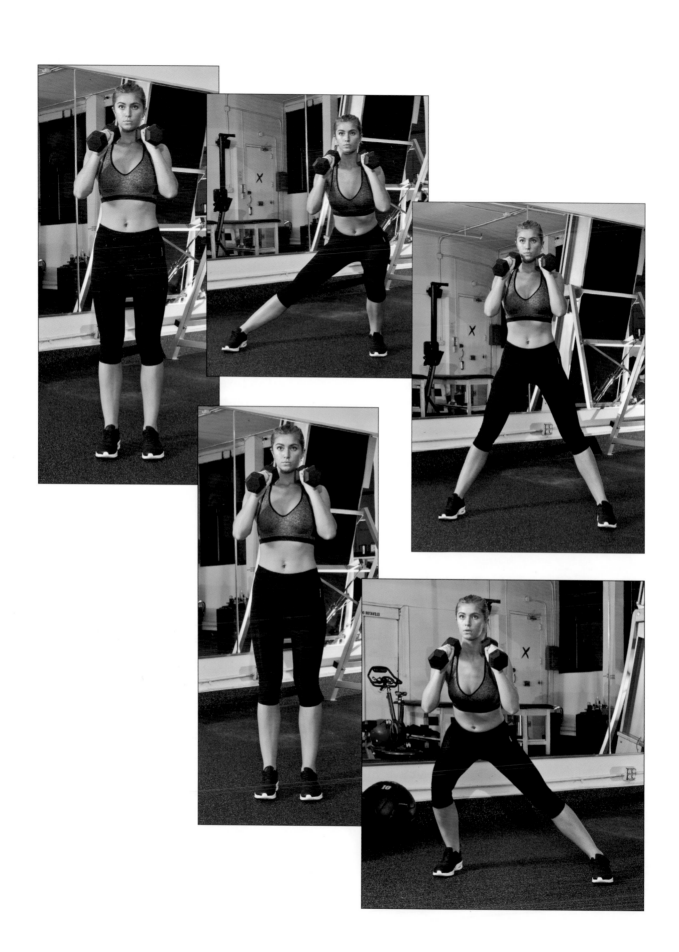

INTRINSIC STRENGTH TRAINING

REPLACEMENT EXERCISE FOR
HACK SQUAT
IST: ALTERNATING REAR STEP HIP HINGE

BOS - bilateral start position - back facing - alternating rear step with hip hinge
POR - ankle height - bilateral hand grip holding both resistance handles at shoulder height

1. Set up with a bilateral stance facing away from the resistance point at ankle height.
2. Hold both resistance handle at the shoulder with both hands.
3. Perform all three phases of IST with each rep: dynamic acceleration, global repetition, and dynamic deceleration.
4. (Dynamic Acceleration) - Take a rear step with the same side as resistance handle— towards the the resistance (BOS)— while simultaneously lowering the but towards the resistance point (POR).
5. (Global Repetition) - Remain in this stance (one foot rear step) and execute one complete hip hinge squat by raising back into a standing position and lowering the torso back down towards the resistance point .(POR)
6. (Dynamic Deceleration) - Return to the bilateral starting position (BOS) while standing upright (POR)
7. Repeat by stepping the opposite foot behind the body.

ANGELO'S ADVICE

1. Leave the majority of the bodies weight on the non stepping leg
2. Focus on challenging the butt to sit behind the ankles - keeping the tension in the powerful muscles and out of the knees.
3. Focus on using your entire body for this exercise.
4. Allow the ankles, knees, hips, and shoulders to move as needed for full body muscle activation —but with precise control during each part of the exercise.
5. Actively press the forefoot and big toe of the non stepping leg into the ground - Activating and stabilizing the entire core to maintain body control, balance, and alignment.
6. Be sure to keep a strong and erect posture by applying tension throughout the core, keeping the spine and head in an neutral position.

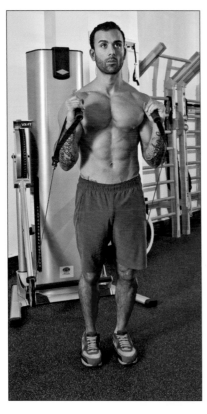 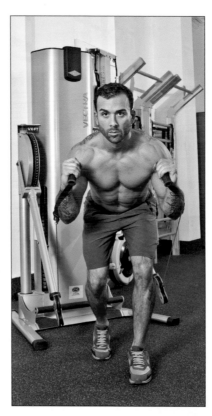 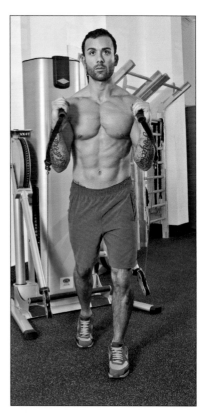

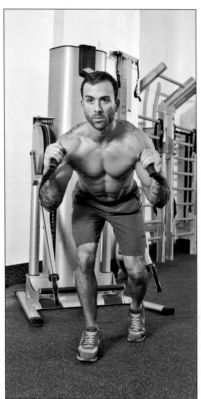 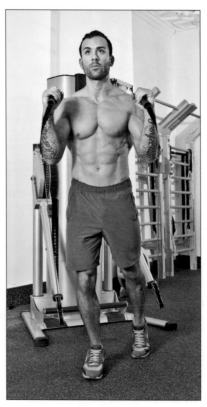

Articulating Arms

The arms must fluidly adapt to the many possible positions of the body, and likewise, the body must also adapt to the many positions of the arms. The arms effect the position of the shoulders and core, which effect how the legs move. Don't let a stationary, limited approach to bicep and triceps training also limit the overall functioning of your body. You can also "pack more heat for the gun show" with the full-body approach of IST.

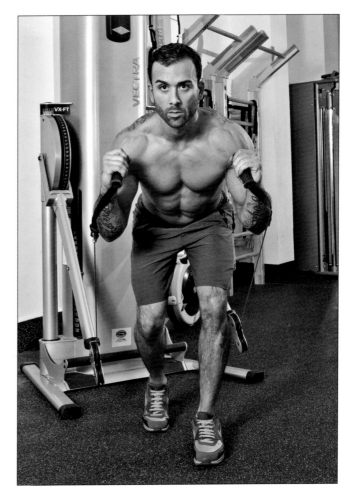

REPLACEMENT EXERCISE FOR SEATED CURL
IST: ALTERNATING FORWARD STEP WITH TWO ARM BICEP CURL

BOS - bilateral start position - forward facing - alternating forward step
POR - hip height - two hands holding hand weight - bicep curl

1. Set up with a bilateral stance while holding a hand weight at hip height with two hand.
2. Perform all three phases of IST with each rep: dynamic acceleration, global repetition, and dynamic deceleration.
3. (Dynamic Acceleration) Take a forward step away from the start position (BOS)—while simultaneously curling both arms directly upward bringing the hands towards the shoulder. (POR).
4. (Global Repetition) Remain in this stance (forward step) and execute one complete bicep curl by lowering the arm back to the hip and curling to the shoulder again (POR).
5. (Dynamic Deceleration) Return back to the bilateral starting position (BOS) while bringing the resistance (POR) back to hip height.
6. Repeat by stepping forward with the opposite foot.

ANGELO'S ADVICE

1. Focus on using your entire body for this exercise.
2. Allow the ankles, knees, hips, and shoulders to move as needed for full body muscle activation—but with precise control during each part of the exercise.
3. Actively press the forefoot and big toe of the rear leg into the ground—activating and stabilizing the entire core to maintain body control, balance, and alignment.
4. Focus on using the entire body for this exercise.
5. Allow the ankles, knees, hips, and shoulders to move as needed—but with precise control during each part of the exercise for full body muscle activation.
6. Be sure to keep a strong and erect posture by applying tension throughout the core, keeping the spine and head in a neutral position.

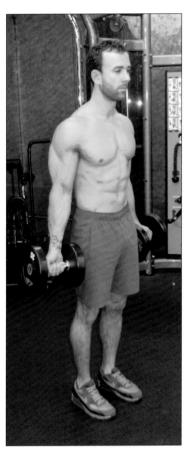
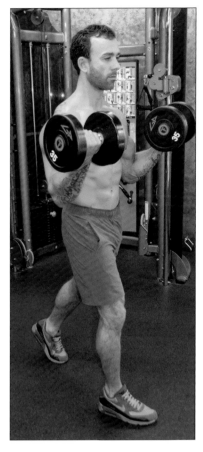
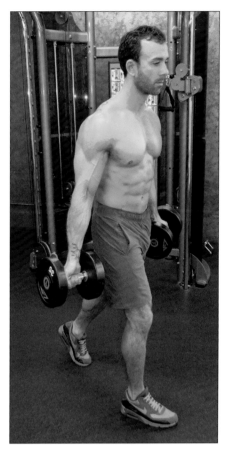
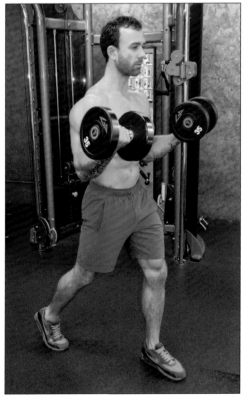
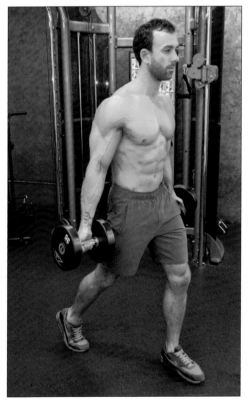

REPLACEMENT EXERCISE FOR PREACHER CURL
IST: ALTERNATING SIDE STEP ONE ARM BICEP CURL TO FOREHEAD

BOS - bilateral start position - front facing - alternating side step
POR - cable - shoulder height - one arm bicep curl to forehead

1. Set up with a bilateral stance while facing the resistance point at shoulder height.
2. Hold a resistance handle with one hand.
3. Perform all three phases of IST with each rep: dynamic acceleration, global repetition, and dynamic deceleration.
4. Take a side step with the foot opposite of the working arm (BOS) while simultaneously curling the resistance handle to the towards the shoulder at head height (POR).
5. (Global Repetition) Remain in this stance (side step) and execute one complete bicep curl, extending the arms down, then curling the resistance handle back towards the shoulder again (POR).
6. (Dynamic Deceleration) Return back to the bilateral starting position (BOS) while bringing the resistance (POR) back to the starting position.
7. Repeat by stepping the opposite foot to the opposite side.

ANGELO'S ADVICE

1. Focus on using your entire body for this exercise.
2. Allow the ankles, knees, hips, and shoulders to move as needed for full body muscle activation—but with precise control during each part of the exercise.
3. Actively press the forefoot and big toe of the non stepping leg into the ground—activating and stabilizing the entire core to maintain body control, balance, and alignment.
4. Actively press down with entire foot of the leg which is transferring the weight. (This leg has a bending knee and active glutes.)
5. Focus on using your entire body for this exercise.
6. Keep your head in a forward-facing, neutral position.

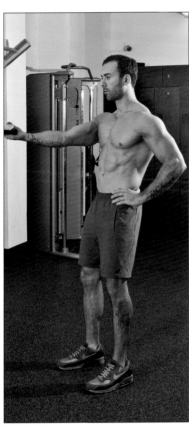
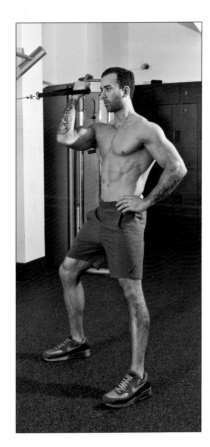
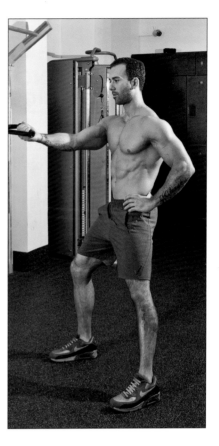
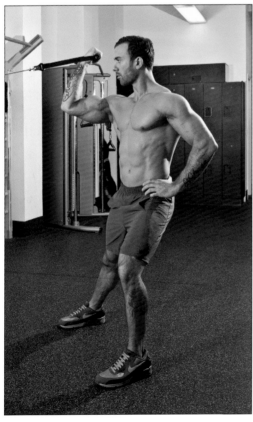
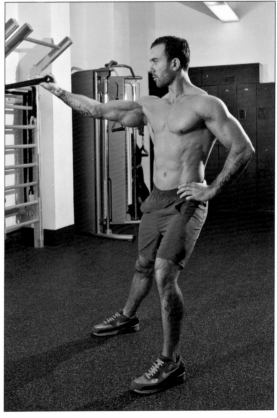

REPLACEMENT EXERCISE FOR
SEATED INCLINE CURL
IST: ALTERNATING FORWARD STEP
WITH INCLINE BICEP CURL

BOS - bilateral starting position - back facing - alternating forward step
POR - cable - hip height - one arm bicep curl to armpit

1. Set up with a bilateral stance with your back facing the resistance point set at hip height.
2. Hold a resistance handle with one hand.
3. Perform all three phases of IST with each rep: dynamic acceleration, global repetition, and dynamic deceleration.
4. Take a forward step with the foot opposite of the working arm (BOS) while simultaneously curling the resistance handle directly forward towards shoulder height (POR).
5. (Global Repetition) Remain in this stance (forward step) and execute one complete bicep curl, extending the arm down, then curling the resistance handle back towards the shoulder again (POR).
6. (Dynamic Deceleration) Return back to the bilateral starting position (BOS) while bringing the resistance (POR) back to the starting position.
7. Repeat by stepping the opposite foot forward.

ANGELO'S ADVICE

1. Focus on using your entire body for this exercise.
2. Allow the ankles, knees, hips, and shoulders to move as needed for full body muscle activation—but with precise control during each part of the exercise.
3. Actively press the forefoot and big toe of the non stepping leg into the ground—activating and stabilizing the entire core to maintain body control, balance, and alignment.
4. Actively press down with entire foot of the leg which is transferring the weight. (This leg has a bending knee and active glutes.)
5. Keep your head in a forward-facing, neutral position.

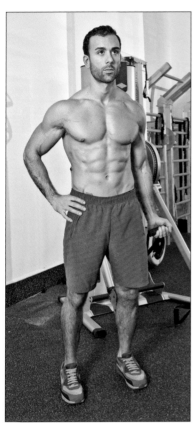
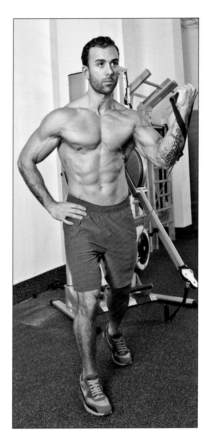
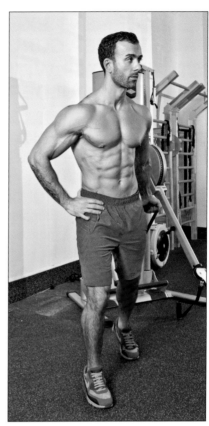
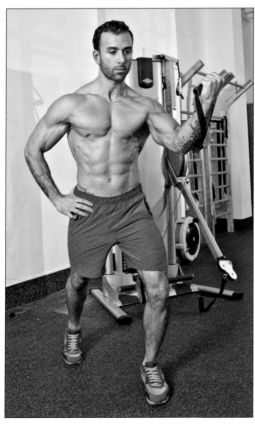
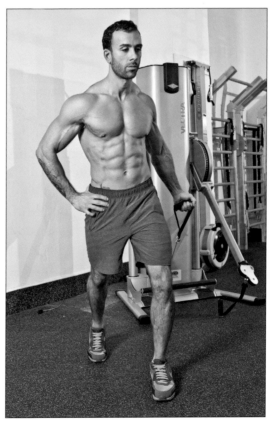

REPLACEMENT EXERCISE FOR
FRONT BICEP CURL
IST: SIDE STEP WITH ONE ARM BICEP CURL (ABOVE SHOULDER)

BOS - bilateral start position - side facing - side step
POR - cable - shoulder height - one arm curl to top of shoulder

1. Set up with a bilateral stance side facing the resistance point set at shoulder height.
2. Hold a resistance handle with the hand closest to the resistance point
3. Perform all three phases of IST with each rep: dynamic acceleration, global repetition, and dynamic deceleration.
4. Take a side step away from the resistance point with the foot furthest from resistance point. (BOS) while simultaneously curling the resistance handle directly towards the shoulder (POR).
5. (Global Repetition) Remain in this stance (side step) and execute one complete bicep curl, extending the arm down, then curling the resistance handle back towards the shoulder again (POR).
6. (Dynamic Deceleration) Return back to the bilateral starting position (BOS) while bringing the resistance (POR) back to the starting position.
7. Repeat for the number of repetitions required by your program.

ANGELO'S ADVICE

1. Challenge more of the upper body by keeping the elbow at shoulder height.
2. Focus on using your entire body for this exercise.
3. Allow the ankles, knees, hips, and shoulders to move as needed for full body muscle activation—but with precise control during each part of the exercise.
4. Actively press down with the entire foot of the leg which is transferring the weight. (This leg has a bending knee and active glutes).
5. Actively press the forefoot and big toe of the non stepping leg into the ground—activating and stabilizing the entire core to maintain body control, balance, and alignment.
6. Keep your head in a forward-facing, neutral position.

Another great variation is a rear rotation step with the opposite foot of the resistance.

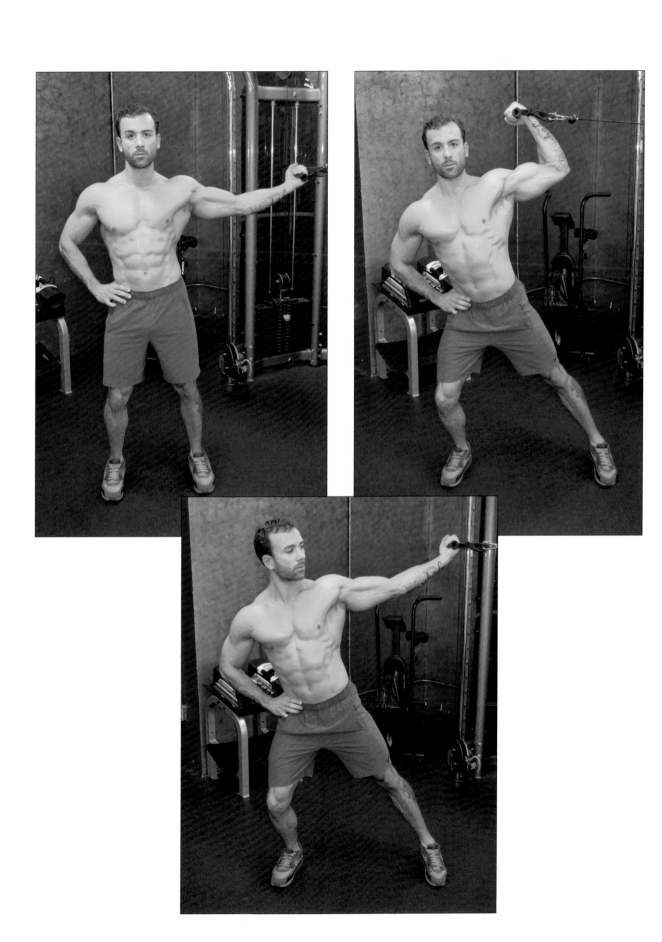

REPLACEMENT EXERCISE FOR
FRONT BICEP CURL
IST: REAR ROTATION STEP
WITH ONE ARM BICEP CURL TO CHEST

BOS - bilateral start position - front facing - rear rotation step
POR - cable - shoulder height - one arm curl to front of shoulder

1. Set up with a bilateral stance front facing the resistance point set at shoulder height.
2. Hold a resistance handle with one hand closest to the resistance point.
3. Perform all three phases of IST with each rep: dynamic acceleration, global repetition, and dynamic deceleration.
4. Take a rear rotation step away from the resistance point with the opposite hand holding the resistance handle (BOS) while simultaneously curling the arm, bringing the handle in front of the chest at shoulder height (POR).
5. (Global Repetition) Remain in this stance (rear rotation step) and execute one complete bicep curl, extending the arm down, then curling the resistance handle back in front of the shoulder again (POR).
6. (Dynamic Deceleration) Return back to the bilateral starting position (BOS) while bringing the resistance (POR) back to the starting position.
7. Repeat for the number of repetitions required by your program.

ANGELO'S ADVICE

1. Challenge more of the upper body by keeping the elbow at shoulder height by actively create tension through the rear shoulder.
2. Focus on using your entire body for this exercise.
3. Allow the ankles, knees, hips, and shoulders to move as needed for full body muscle activation—but with precise control during each part of the exercise.
4. Actively press down with the entire foot of the stepping leg which is transferring the weight. (This leg has a bending knee and active glutes).
5. Actively press the forefoot and big toe of the non stepping leg into the ground—pivot this foot as needed to remain body control, balance, and alignment.
6. Keep your head in a forward-facing, neutral position.

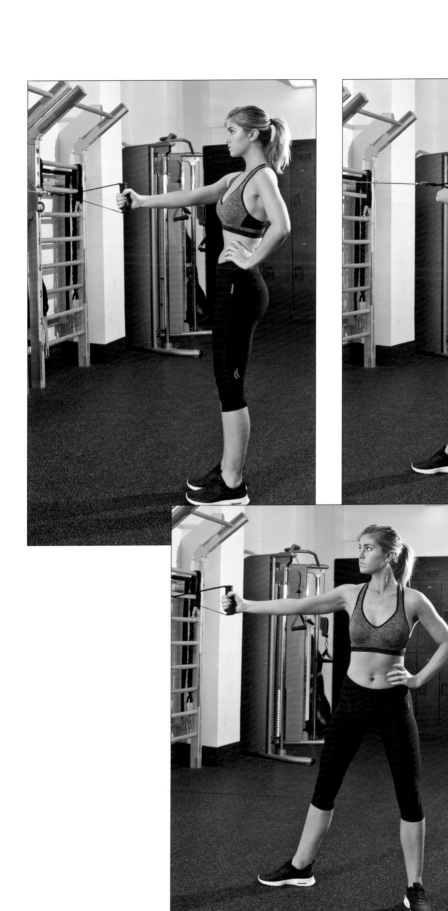

REPLACEMENT EXERCISE FOR
HAMMER CURL
IST: ALTERNATING REAR ROTATION STEP
WITH ROPE CURL

BOS - bilateral start position - forward facing - rear rotation step
POR - cable - ankle height - bilateral bicep curl to shoulder height
same side of body rotation

1.   Set up with a bilateral stance while facing the resistance point at ankle height.
2.   Hold one resistance handle in each hand.
3.   Perform all three phases of IST with each rep: dynamic acceleration, global repetition, and dynamic deceleration.
4.   Take a rear rotation step away from the resistance point (BOS) while simultaneously curling both arms to the same side shoulder (POR).
5.   (Global Repetition) Remain in this stance (rear rotation step) and execute one complete bicep curl, extending the arm down, then curling the resistance handles back in front of the shoulder again (POR).
6.   (Dynamic Deceleration) Return back to the bilateral starting position (BOS) while bringing the resistance (POR) back to the starting position.
7.   Repeat by taking a rear rotation step with the opposite side foot.

ANGELO'S ADVICE

1.   Focus on using your entire body for this exercise.
2.   Allow the ankles, knees, hips, and shoulders to move as needed for full body muscle activation—but with precise control during each part of the exercise.
3.   Actively press down with the entire foot of the stepping leg which is transferring the weight. (This leg has a bending knee and active glutes).
4.   Actively press the forefoot and big toe of the non stepping leg into the ground—pivot this foot as needed to remain body control, balance, and alignment.
5.   Keep your eyes on the resistance handle to ensure core rotation.

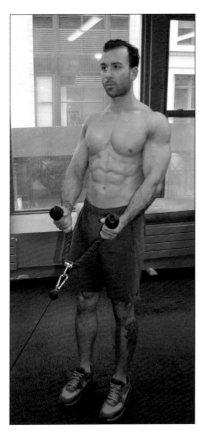
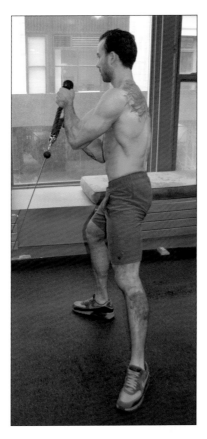
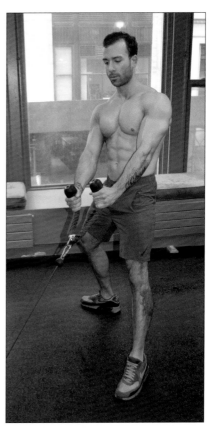
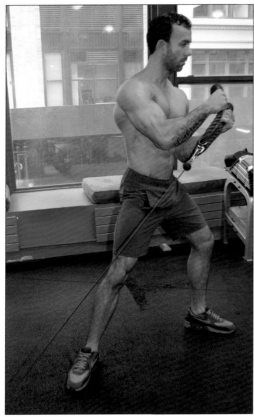
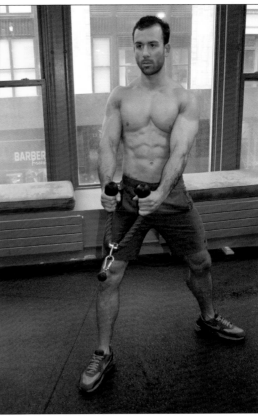

REPLACEMENT EXERCISE FOR TRICEPS PUSH DOWN
IST: ALTERNATING REAR STEP WITH CABLE PUSH DOWNS

BOS - bilateral start position - forward facing - alternating rear step
POR - cable - shoulder height - two arm triceps extensions to hip

1. Set up with a bilateral stance front facing the resistance point set at shoulder height.
2. Hold a resistance handle with both hands.
3. Perform all three phases of IST with each rep: dynamic acceleration, global repetition, and dynamic deceleration.
4. Take a rear step away from the resistance point with both hands holding the resistance handles (BOS) while simultaneously extending the triceps, pushing the handles down to the hips (POR).
5. (Global Repetition) Remain in this stance (rear step) and execute one complete tricep extension, allowing the hands to come back up to shoulder height by bending at the elbow, the extending the arms back down to the hip (POR).
6. (Dynamic Deceleration) Return back to the bilateral starting position (BOS) while bringing the resistance (POR) back to the starting position.
7. Repeat by taking a rear step with the opposite foot.

ANGELO'S ADVICE

1. Focus on using your entire body for this exercise.
2. Allow the ankles, knees, hips, and shoulders to move as needed for full body muscle activation—but with precise control during each part of the exercise.
3. Actively press down with the entire foot of the non stepping leg which is transferring the weight. (This leg has a bending knee and active glutes).
4. Actively press the forefoot and big toe of the stepping leg into the ground to remain body control, balance, and alignment.
5. Keep your head in a forward-facing, neutral position.

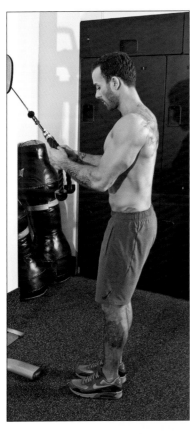
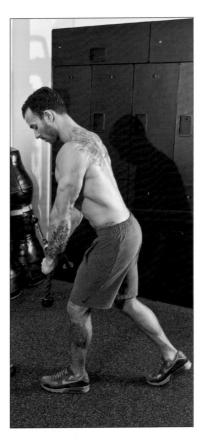
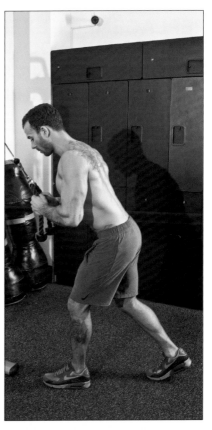
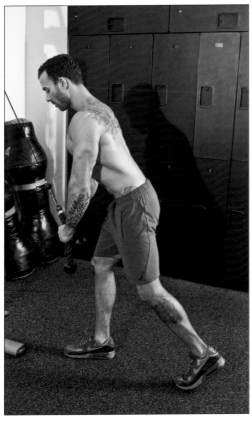
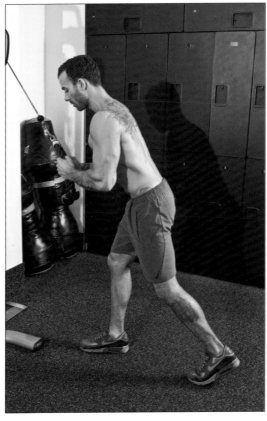

REPLACEMENT EXERCISE FOR TRICEPS PUSH DOWN
IST: ALTERNATING SIDE STEP WITH CABLE PUSH DOWNS

BOS - bilateral start position - forward facing - alternating side step
POR - cable - shoulder height - triceps extension to hip

1. Set up with a bilateral stance front facing the resistance point set at shoulder height.
2. Hold a resistance handle with one hand.
3. Perform all three phases of IST with each rep: dynamic acceleration, global repetition, and dynamic deceleration.
4. Take a side step away from the resistance point with one hand holding the resistance handle. (BOS) while simultaneously extending the triceps, pushing the handle down to the hip (POR).
5. (Global Repetition) Remain in this stance (side step) and execute one complete tricep extension, allowing the hands to come back up to shoulder height by bending at the elbow, the extending the arm back down to the hip (POR).
6. (Dynamic Deceleration) Return back to the bilateral starting position (BOS) while bringing the resistance (POR) back to the starting position.
7. Repeat by taking a side step to the opposite side with the opposite foot.

ANGELO'S ADVICE

1. Focus on using your entire body for this exercise.
2. Let the change of body position change the angle of tricep tension.
3. Allow the ankles, knees, hips, and shoulders to move as needed for full body muscle activation—but with precise control during each part of the exercise.
4. Actively press down with the entire foot of the stepping leg which is transferring the weight. (This leg has a bending knee and active glutes).
5. Actively press the forefoot and big toe of the non stepping leg into the ground to remain body control, balance, and alignment.
6. Keep your head in a forward-facing, neutral position.

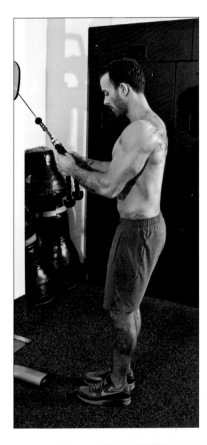
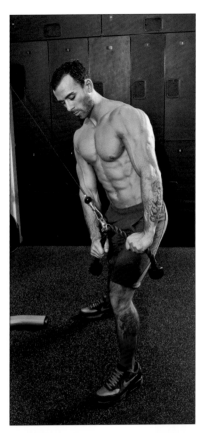
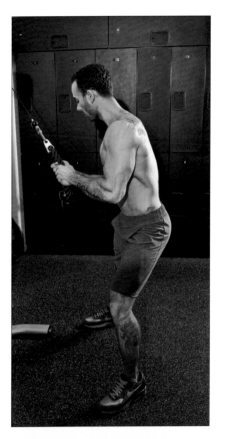
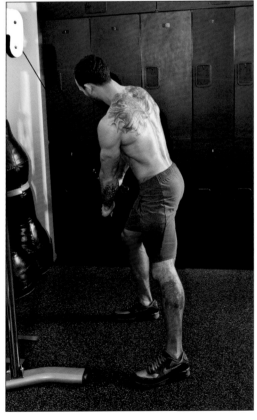
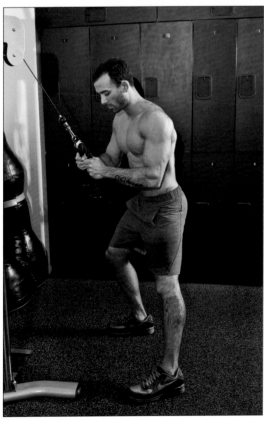

REPLACEMENT EXERCISE FOR REVERSE GRIP PUSH DOWN
IST: REAR ROTATION TRICEPS UNDERHAND GRIP PUSH DOWN

BOS - bilateral start position - forward facing - rear rotation step
POR - cable - shoulder height - unilateral underhand grip triceps extension to hip

1. Set up with a bilateral stance front facing the resistance point set at shoulder height.
2. Hold a resistance handle with one hand - with the palm facing upward.
3. Perform all three phases of IST with each rep: dynamic acceleration, global repetition, and dynamic deceleration.
4. Take a rear rotation step away from the resistance point with the same side hand holding the resistance handle (BOS) while simultaneously extending the tricep, pulling the handle down to the hip (POR).
5. (Global Repetition) Remain in this stance (rear rotation step) and execute one complete tricep extension, allowing the hand to come back up to shoulder height by bending at the elbow, the extending the arm back down to the hip (POR).
6. (Dynamic Deceleration) Return back to the bilateral starting position (BOS) while bringing the resistance (POR) back to the starting position.
7. Repeat for the number of repetitions required by your program.

ANGELO'S ADVICE

1. Focus on using your entire body for this exercise.
2. Let the change of body position change the angle of tricep tension.
3. Allow the ankles, knees, hips, and shoulders to move as needed for full body muscle activation—but with precise control during each part of the exercise.
4. Actively press down with the entire foot of the stepping leg which is transferring the weight. (This leg has a bending knee and active glutes).
5. Actively press the forefoot and big toe of the non stepping leg into the ground to remain body control, balance, and alignment (pivot if necessary).
6. Keep your head in a forward-facing, neutral position.

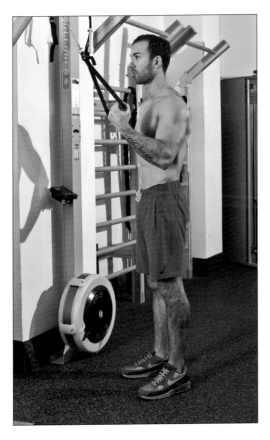
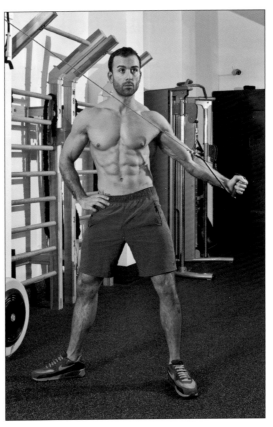
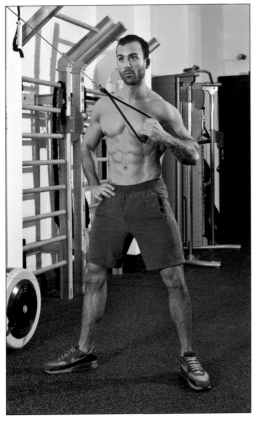
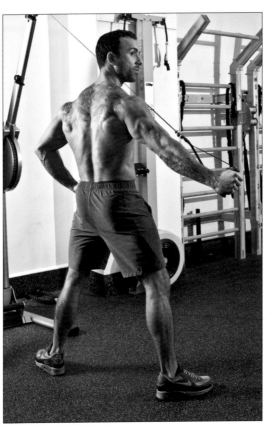

REPLACEMENT EXERCISE FOR TRICEPS KICKBACKS
IST: ALTERNATING REAR STEP ONE ARM TRICEPS KICKBACKS

BOS - bilateral start position - back facing - alternating forward step
POR - cable - shoulder height - one arm overhead tricep extension

1. Set up with a bilateral stance back facing the resistance point set at shoulder height.
2. Hold a resistance handle with one hand.
3. Perform all three phases of IST with each rep: dynamic acceleration, global repetition, and dynamic deceleration.
4. Take a forward step away from the resistance point with the same side hand holding the resistance handle (BOS) while simultaneously extending the tricep overhead (POR).
5. (Global Repetition) Remain in this stance (forward step) and execute one complete tricep extension, allowing the hand to come back up to shoulder height by bending at the elbow, the extending the arm overhead again (POR).
6. (Dynamic Deceleration) Return back to the bilateral starting position (BOS) while bringing the resistance (POR) back to the starting position.
7. Repeat by stepping the opposite leg forward.

ANGELO'S ADVICE

1. Focus on using your entire body for this exercise.
2. Allow the ankles, knees, hips, and shoulders to move as needed for full body muscle activation—but with precise control during each part of the exercise.
3. Actively press down with the entire foot of the stepping leg which is transferring the weight. (This leg has a bending knee and active glutes).
4. Actively press the forefoot and big toe of the non stepping leg into the ground to remain body control, balance, and alignment.
5. Keep your head in a forward-facing, neutral position.

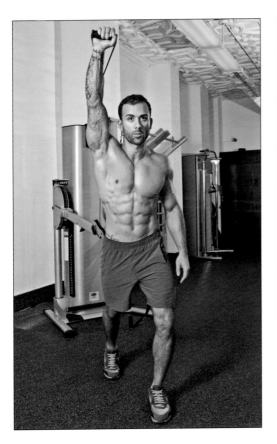
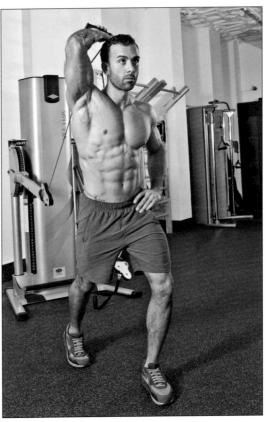
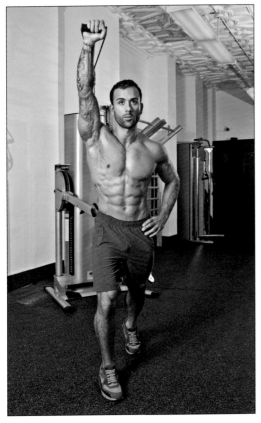
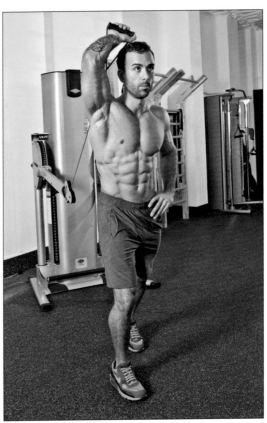

REPLACEMENT EXERCISE FOR TRICEPS KICKBACKS
IST: ALTERNATING REAR STEP ONE ARM TRICEPS KICKBACKS

BOS - bilateral start position - forward facing - alternating rear step
POR - cable - hip height - unilateral triceps extension

1. Set up with a bilateral stance front facing the resistance point set at hip height.
2. Hold a resistance handle with one hand.
3. Perform all three phases of IST with each rep: dynamic acceleration, global repetition, and dynamic deceleration.
4. Take a rear step away from the resistance point with the same side hand holding the resistance handle (BOS) while simultaneously extending the tricep, pushing the handle down to the hip (POR).
5. (Global Repetition) Remain in this stance (rear step) and execute one complete tricep extension, allowing the hand to come back up to shoulder height by bending at the elbow, the extending the arm back down to the hip (POR).
6. (Dynamic Deceleration) Return back to the bilateral starting position (BOS) while bringing the resistance (POR) back to the starting position.
7. Repeat by stepping the opposite foot backwards.

ANGELO'S ADVICE

1. Focus on using your entire body for this exercise.
2. Let the change of body position change the angle of tricep tension.
3. Allow the ankles, knees, hips, and shoulders to move as needed for full body muscle activation —but with precise control during each part of the exercise.
4. Actively press down with the entire foot of the non stepping leg which is transferring the weight. (This leg has a bending knee and active glutes).
5. Actively press the forefoot and big toe of the stepping leg into the ground to remain body control, balance, and alignment. (pivot if necessary).
6. Keep your head in a forward-facing, neutral position.

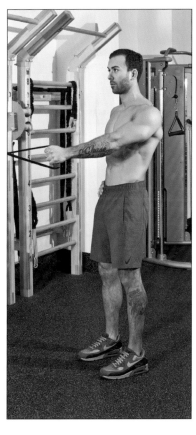 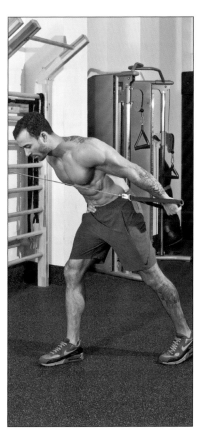 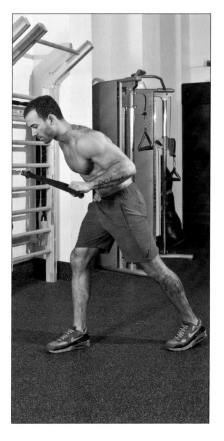

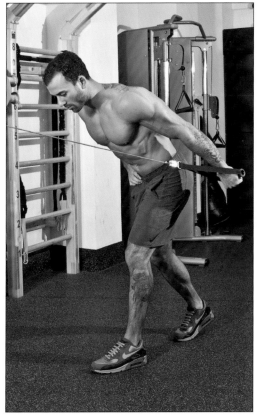 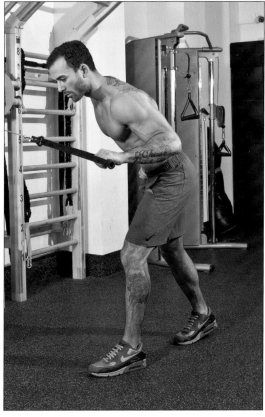

REPLACEMENT EXERCISE FOR LYING TRICEPS SKULL CRUSHERS
IST: ALTERNATING REAR ROTATION STEP TRICEPS CRUSHERS

BOS - bilateral start position - back facing - alternating rear rotation step
POR - cable - shoulder height - two arm triceps extension in front of the head

1. Set up with a bilateral stance back facing the resistance point set at shoulder height.
2. Hold the resistance handles with two hands.
3. Perform all three phases of IST with each rep: dynamic acceleration, global repetition, and dynamic deceleration.
4. Take a rear rotation step towards the resistance point (BOS) while simultaneously extending the triceps, pushing the handles away from the body at above shoulder height (POR).
5. (Global Repetition) Remain in this stance (rear rotation step) and execute one complete tricep extension, allowing the hands to come back up to shoulder by bending at the elbow, then extending the arms back away from the body at above shoulder height (POR).
6. (Dynamic Deceleration) Return back to the bilateral starting position (BOS) while bringing the resistance (POR) back to the starting position.
7. Repeat by taking a rear rotation step to the opposite side with the opposite leg.

ANGELO'S ADVICE

1. Focus on using your entire body for this exercise
2. Let the change of body position change the angle of tricep tension.
3. Allow the ankles, knees, hips, and shoulders to move as needed for full body muscle activation—but with precise control during each part of the exercise.
4. Actively press down with the entire foot of the stepping leg which is transferring the weight. (This leg has a bending knee and active glutes).
5. Actively press the forefoot and big toe of the non stepping leg into the ground—pivot this leg and foot as necessary for body control, balance, and alignment.
6. Keep your head in a forward-facing, neutral position.

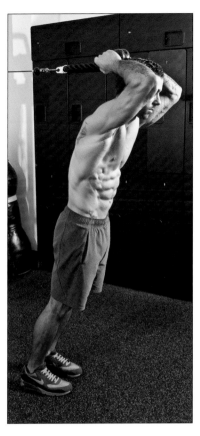
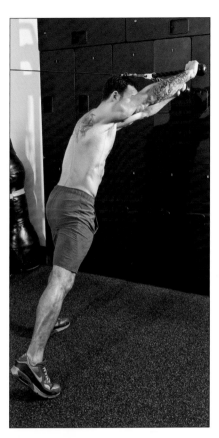
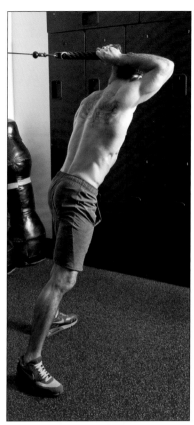

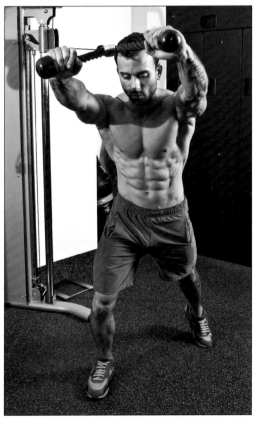
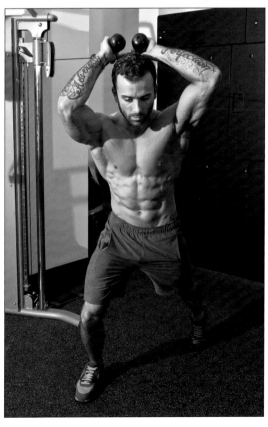

REPLACEMENT EXERCISE FOR
SIDE TRICEPS EXTENSION
IST: SIDE STEP ACROSS BODY TRICEPS EXTENSION

BOS - bilateral start position - side facing - side step
POR - cable - shoulder height - one arm triceps extension away from the body

1. Set up with a bilateral stance side facing the resistance point set at shoulder height.
2. Hold the resistance handle with the hand furthest from the point of resistance.
3. Perform all three phases of IST with each rep: dynamic acceleration, global repetition, and dynamic deceleration.
4. Take a side step away from the resistance point (BOS) while simultaneously extending the triceps, pushing the handle away from the body and resistance point at above shoulder height (POR).
5. (Global Repetition) Remain in this stance (side step) and execute one complete tricep extension, allowing the hand to come back to the front of the shoulder by bending at the elbow, then extending the arm back away from the body at shoulder height (POR).
6. (Dynamic Deceleration) Return back to the bilateral starting position (BOS) while bringing the resistance (POR) back to the starting position.
7. Repeat for the number of repetitions required by your program.

ANGELO'S ADVICE

1. Focus on using your entire body for this exercise.
2. Challenge more of the upper body by keeping the elbow at shoulder height by actively create tension through the rear shoulder.
3. Allow the ankles, knees, hips, and shoulders to move as needed for full body muscle activation —but with precise control during each part of the exercise.
4. Actively press down with the entire foot of the stepping leg which is transferring the weight. (This leg has a bending knee and active glutes).
5. Actively press the forefoot and big toe of the non stepping leg into the ground—pivot this leg and foot as necessary for body control, balance, and alignment.
6. Keep your head in a forward-facing, neutral position.

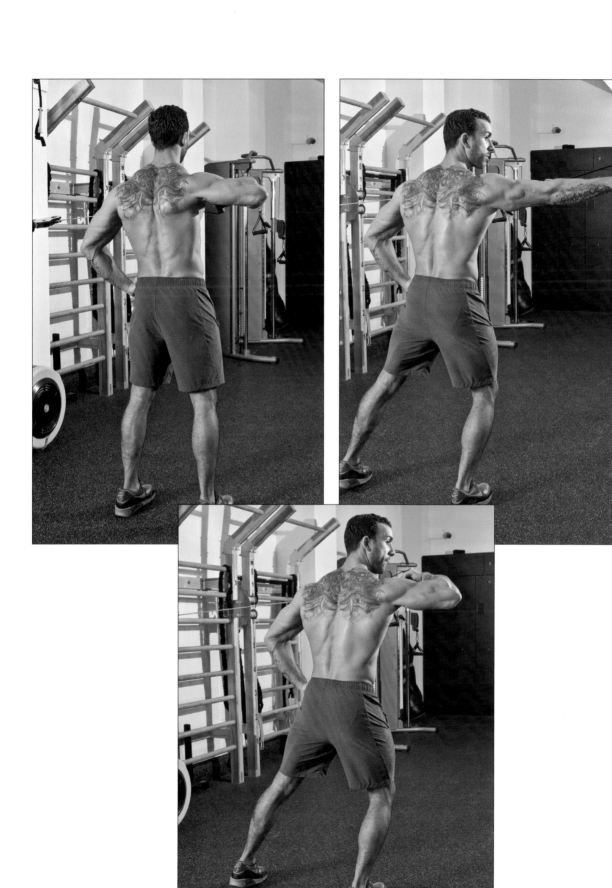

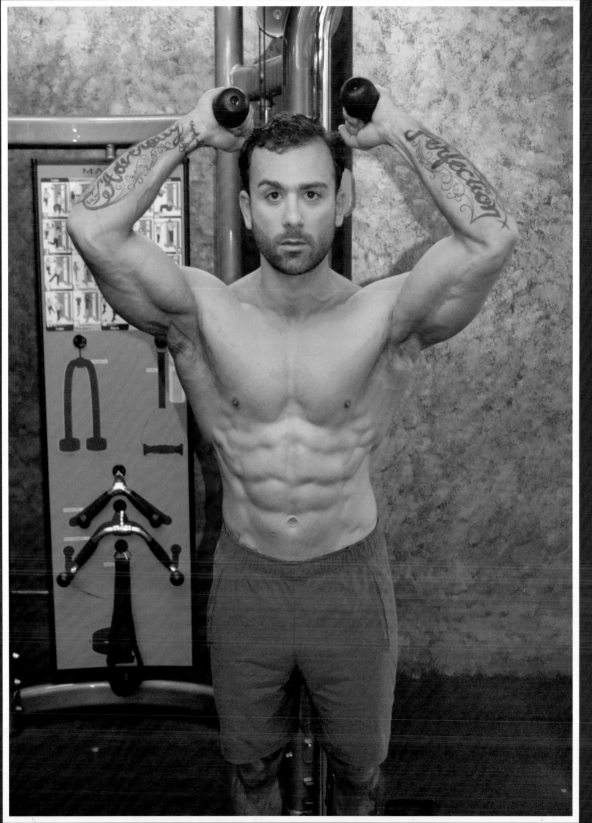

Abdominal Focus

As if focusing on training the extremities doesn't challenge your core enough—enjoy these full body dynamic plank and crunch variations."

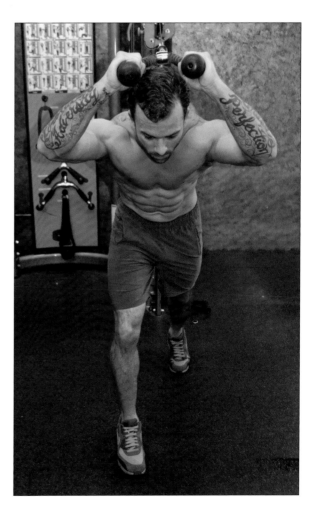

REPLACEMENT EXERCISE FOR
WEIGHTED CRUNCHES
IST: ALTERNATING FORWARD STEP GLOBAL CRUNCH

BOS - bilateral start position - back facing - alternating forward step
POR - cable - shoulder height - both hands at shoulder or overhead -
global flex and extend.

1. Set up with a bilateral stance back facing the resistance point set at shoulder height.
2. Hold the resistance handles with two hands.
3. Perform all three phases of IST with each rep: dynamic acceleration, global repetition, and dynamic deceleration.
4. Take a forward step away from the resistance point (BOS) while simultaneously flexing through the core. Resist the handle tension by pushing the handles with the motion of the body at shoulder height (POR).
5. (Global Repetition) Remain in this stance (forward step) and execute one global "crunch", by flexing the body forward, then controlling the body as we extend back towards the resistance point (POR).
6. (Dynamic Deceleration) Return back to the bilateral starting position (BOS) while bringing the resistance (POR) back to the starting position.
7. Repeat by taking a forward step with the opposite leg.

ANGELO'S ADVICE

1. Focus on using your entire body for this exercise.
2. Let the change of body position change the angle of abdominal focus.
3. Allow the ankles, knees, hips, and shoulders to move as needed for full body muscle activation—but with precise control during each part of the exercise.
4. Actively press down with the entire foot of the stepping leg which is transferring the weight. (This leg has a bending knee and active glutes).
5. Actively press the forefoot and big toe of the non stepping leg into the ground for body control, balance, and alignment.
6. Keep your head in a forward-facing, neutral position.

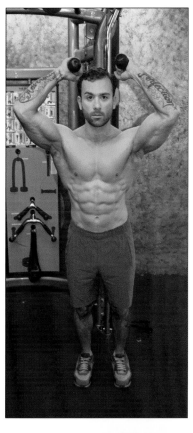
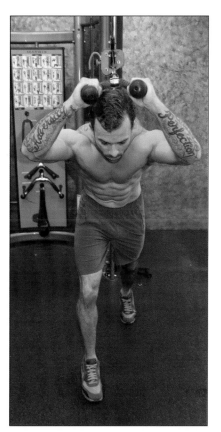
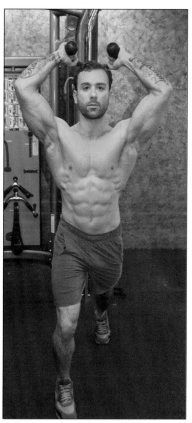
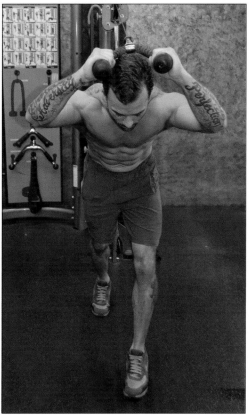
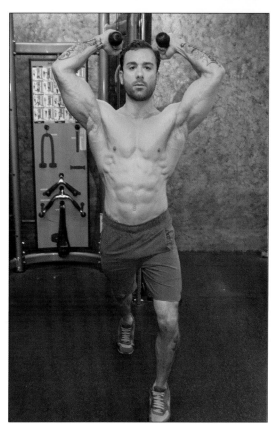

STEPPING VARIATIONS TO STATIC PLANK HOLDS

1. Start with your feet in a bilateral stance, shoulder width apart.
2. Walk both hands out on the floor until the hands are directly underneath of your shoulder.
3. Assume a "plank" position.
4. Proceed with the chosen POR.

ANGELO'S ADVICE

1. Allow every muscle in the body to help with distributing the work load.
2. Actively apply pressure into the ground through your legs and feet to create lower body tension.
3. Actively apply pressure into the ground through your shoulders and fingers to create upper body tension.
4. This extremity tension will radiate through the core—ensuring core tension and more muscular activation.

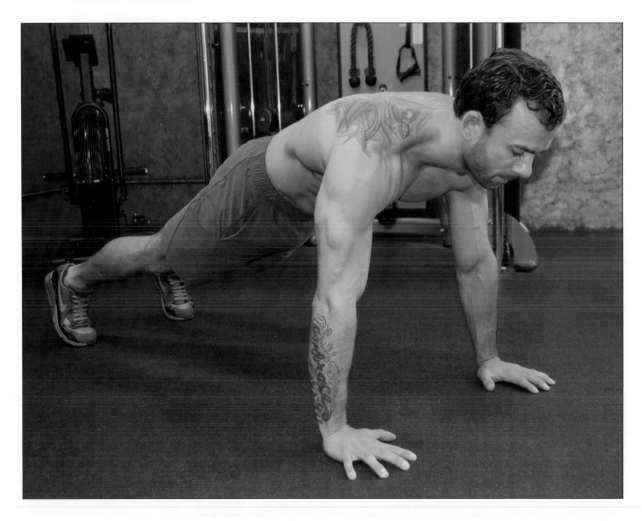

IST: FORWARD HAND STEP PLANK

BOS - bilateral hands and feet - plank position
POR - alternating forward hand step placement

ANGELO'S ADVICE

1. Allow every muscle in the body to help with distributing the work load.
2. Actively apply pressure into the ground through your legs and feet to create lower body tension.
3. Actively apply pressure into the ground through your shoulders and fingers to create upper body tension.
4. This extremity tension will radiate through the core—ensuring core tension and more muscular activation.
5. Allow for more of the body's weight to shift into the stepping hand.

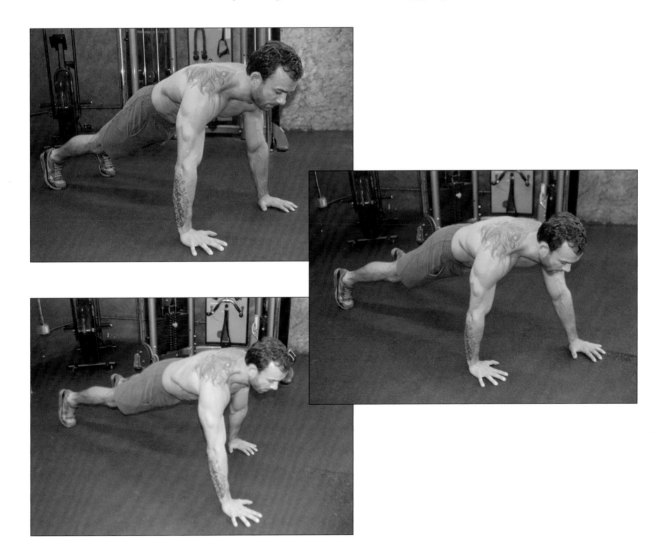

IST: SIDE HAND STEP PLANK

BOS - bilateral hands and feet - plank position
POR - alternating side hand step placement

ANGELO'S ADVICE

1. Allow every muscle in the body to help with distributing the work load.
2. Actively apply pressure into the ground through your legs and feet to create lower body tension.
3. Actively apply pressure into the ground through your shoulders and fingers to create upper body tension.
4. This extremity tension will radiate through the core - ensuring core tension and more muscular activation.
5. allow for more of the body's weight to shift into the stepping hand.

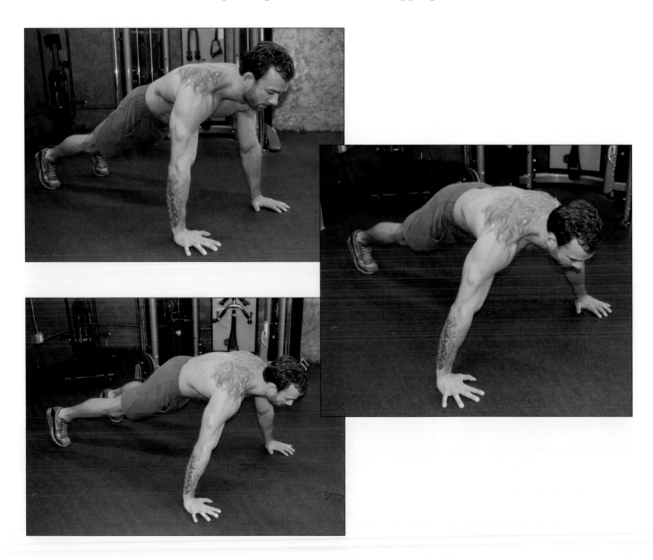

INTRINSIC STRENGTH TRAINING

IST: REAR ROTATION HAND PLANK

BOS - bilateral hands and feet - plank position
POR - alternating rear rotational hand placement

ANGELO'S ADVICE

1. Allow every muscle in the body to help with distributing the work load.
2. Actively apply pressure into the ground through your legs and feet to create lower body tension.
3. Actively apply pressure into the ground through your shoulders and fingers to create upper body tension.
4. This extremity tension will radiate through the core—ensuring core tension and more muscular activation.
5. Allow for more of the body's weight to shift into the stepping hand.

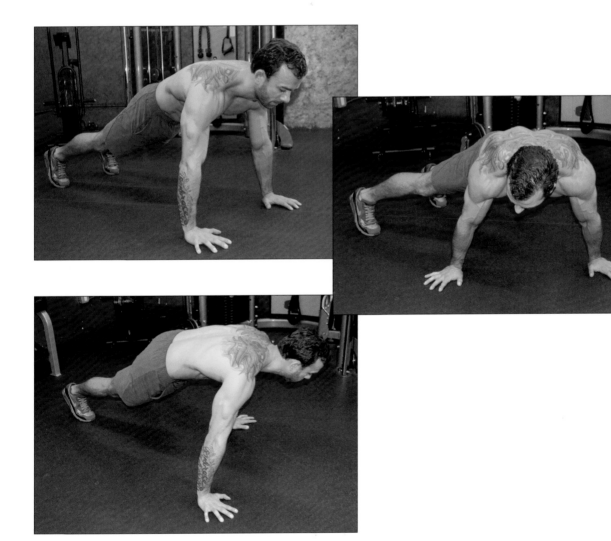

IST: SIDE FOOT STEP PLANK

BOS - bilateral hands and feet - plank position
POR - alternating side foot placement

ANGELO'S ADVICE

1. Allow every muscle in the body to help with distributing the work load.
2. Actively apply pressure into the ground through your legs and feet to create lower body tension.
3. Actively apply pressure into the ground through your shoulders and fingers to create upper body tension.
4. This extremity tension will radiate through the core - ensuring core tension and more muscular activation.
5. Allow for more of the body's weight to shift into the stepping foot.

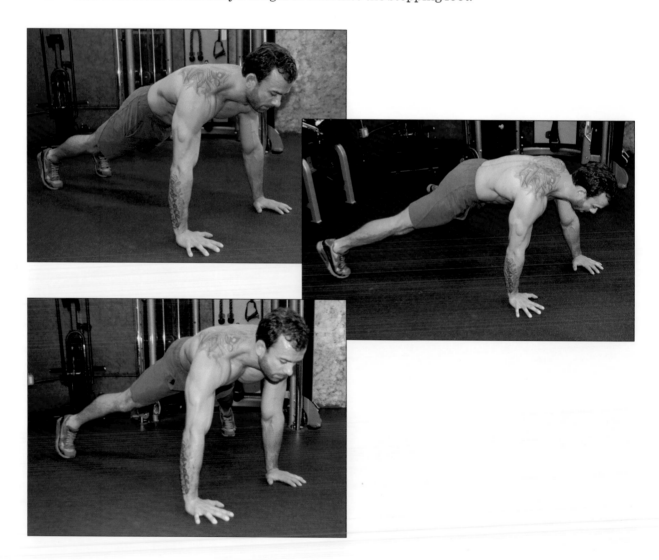

IST: FORWARD STEP PLANK

BOS - bilateral hands and feet - plank position
POR - alternating forward foot placement

ANGELO'S ADVICE

1. Allow every muscle in the body to help with distributing the work load.
2. Actively apply pressure into the ground through your legs and feet to create lower body tension.
3. Actively apply pressure into the ground through your shoulders and fingers to create upper body tension.
4. This extremity tension will radiate through the core - ensuring core tension and more muscular activation.
5. Allow for more of the body's weight to shift into the stepping foot.

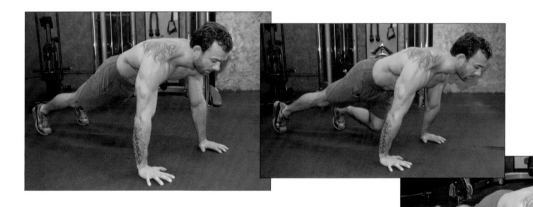

IST: REAR STEP PLANK

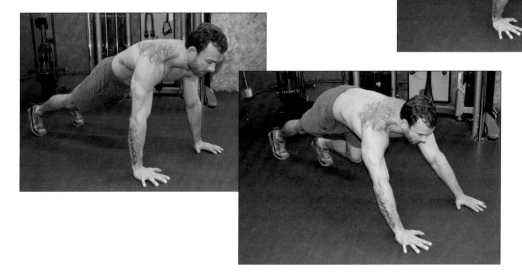

IST: REAR CROSS OVER STEP PLANK

BOS - bilateral hands and feet - plank position
POR - alternating rear cross over foot placement

ANGELO'S ADVICE

1. Allow every muscle in the body to help with distributing the work load.
2. Actively apply pressure into the ground through your legs and feet to create lower body tension.
3. Actively apply pressure into the ground through your shoulders and fingers to create upper body tension.
4. This extremity tension will radiate through the core - ensuring core tension and more muscular activation.
5. Allow for more of the body's weight to shift into the non stepping foot.

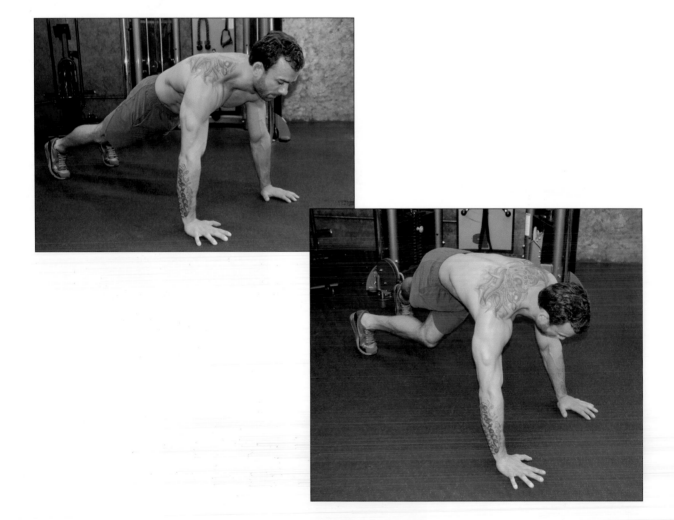

SECTION 5

SAMPLE EXERCISE COMBINATIONS, CIRCUITS, AND WEEKLY WORKOUT SPLITS

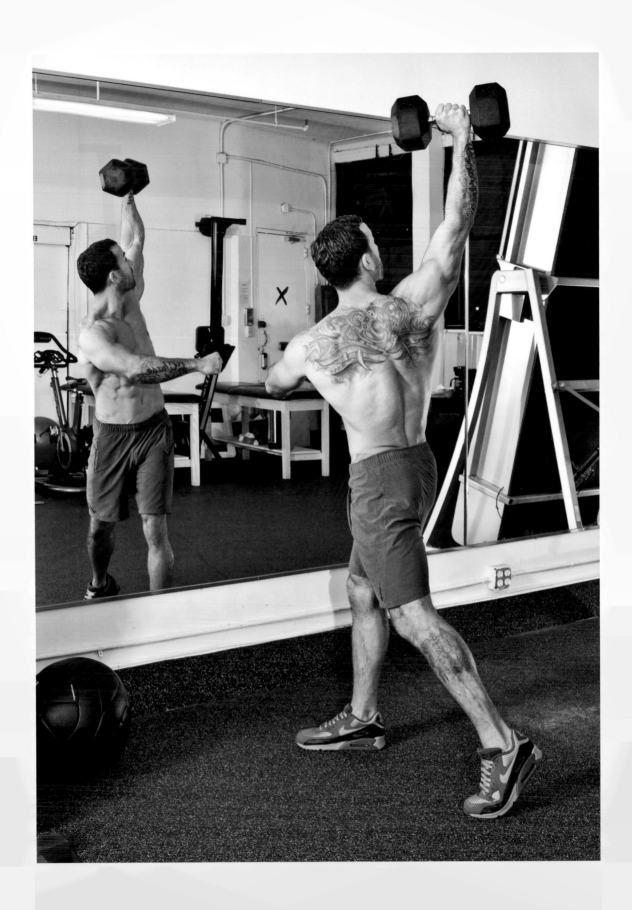

SAMPLE EXERCISE COMBINATIONS

IST Chest Press Step Complex - Shoulder Height - (left hand holding, side set up) right foot side step chest press & left foot forward step chest press

IST Overhead Press Step Complex - Ankle Height - (left hand holding cable) right foot side step overhead bend press & left foot forward step overhead press

IST Cable Row Step Complex - Shoulder Height - (left hand holding cable) left foot rear rotation row & right foot side step row

IST Push & Pull Rotation Complex - Shoulder Height - (left hand holding cable) left foot rear rotation step row & right foot rear rotation step chest press

IST Full Line Row - Hip Height - (left hand holding cable) left rear rotation step row flowing into triceps extension away from body

IST Front Squat Complex - Kettlebell - forward step squat, side step squat, rear step squat, rear rotation step squat

IST Deadlift Complex - Kettlebell - rear step deadlift, rear rotation step deadlift, side step deadlift, forward step deadlift

IST Push Up Complex - 3 in 1 - eyes over left shoulder, eyes facing center, eyes over right shoulder

IST Pull Up Complex - 3 in 1 - eyes over left shoulder, eyes facing center, eyes over right shoulder

IST Hip to Overhead - alternating forward step with one arm dumbbell curl to overhead press

Squat Butt Builder Combo - Hand Weight - right foot side step squat (toe tap) and right foot rear crossover step squat (toe tap)

Post your workouts, moves, results under hash tags

#SpineStrong #Takeyourfirststep #STEPFIRST #IST

#ISTraining #intrinsicstrengthtraining

SAMPLE CIRCUITS

IST Ankle Height Pulley Circuit with Squat Complex
- Front facing - alternating side step row
- Side facing - side step overhead bend press
- Back facing - alternating front step bicep curl
- Front facing - alternating rear step triceps kick back
- Side facing - rear rotation shoulder press
- IST push up - 3 in 1
- Squat complex (alternating rear, rear rotation, and side step)

IST Hip or Shoulder Pulley Circuit with IST Leg Adductor IST Push Up and IST Pull Up
- Front facing - alternating rear step row
- Back facing - alternating forward step chest press
- Side facing - side step triceps extension away from body
- Side facing - side step bicep curl towards body
- IST rear rotation step shoulder rotation press
- IST pull up - 3 in 1
- IST abductor/adductor squat

IST Overhead Pulley Circuit with Deadlift Complex
- Front facing - same side rear rotation step row
- Back facing - alternating rear step decline chest press
- Front facing - alternating side step bicep curl to forehead
- Front facing - alternating forward step overhead triceps extension
- Alternating forward step overhead shoulder press
- Deadlift complex
- IST dips

IST Body Weight Circuit
- IST push up 3 in 1
- IST pull up 3 in 1
- IST squat (forward, rear, side, rotation step (toe tap)
- IST dip 3 in 1
- IST deadlift (alternating rear cross over step, side step, forward step)
- IST leg extension squat

Low and High Circuit

Cable at ankle height - 3x8
- Alternating forward step with one arm row - forward facing set up
- Rear rotation step with curl to shoulder press - side facing set up
- Alternating side step front load squat

Cable at overhead height- 3x8
- Rear rotation step with curl to decline chest press - side facing set up
- Alternating forward step with one arm row - forward facing set up
- Alternating side step deadlift

Hip Height Circuit

- Front facing - rear rotation row to triceps extension
- Side facing - side step bicep curl to chest press across the body
- Rear rotation step and rotating shoulder press
- Leg extension replacement (alternating forward step squat on toes)
- Side set up, side step overhead bend press

Leg Burn Kettlebell or Dumbbell Circuit

Please start with bodyweight only while you learn the movement patterns.

- Squat rear rotation step (kettlebell or dumbbell in hand same side as the stepping foot)
- Deadlift alternating side step toe tap (use two kettlebells or two dumbbells)
- Leg extension replacement (on toe, squat while alternating the forward step, do not use weight until you can complete 20 controlled reps)
- Leg press replacement (rear crossover step squat) kettlebell front racked or goblet hold
- Deadlift alternating rear step (barbell or 2 dumbbells/kettlebells)
- Adductor replacement - alternating side step squat slide (kettlebell or dumbbell in front hold position)
- Rear cross over step deadlift

SAMPLE WEEKLY WORKOUT SPLITS

IST 3 DAY SPLIT
Each exercise should be done for a set of 8-12

POR SHOULDER HEIGHT	POR ANKLE HEIGHT	POR OVERHEAD
IST Alt. Rear Step Row - Front Facing	IST Alt. Side Step 2 Arm Row - Front Facing	IST Rear Rotation Step Tricep Extension - Forward Facing
IST Alt. Forward Step Chest Press - Back Facing	IST Alt. Side Step Overhead Press - Side facing	IST Alt. Side Step Decline Chest Press - Back Facing
IST alt. Side step 2 Arm Tricep Extension to Hip - Side Facing	IST Rear Step Toe Reach Squat	IST Rear Rotation Deadlift
IST Side Step Bicep Curl to Front of Chest - Side Facing	IST Alt Front Step 2 Arm Bicep Curl - Back Facing	IST alt side step bicep curl to forehead - Front facing
IST Rear Rotation Shoulder Rotating Press	IST Rear Rotation Step Squat	IST Alt Forward Step Overhead Tricep Ext - Back Facing
IST Pull Up (3 in 1)	IST Alt Rear Step Tricep Extension to Hip - Front Facing	IST Alt Forward Step Overhead Shoulder Press
IST Alt. Side Squat Slide	IST Side Step Toe Tap Squat	IST Forward Step Deadlift With Barbell
IST Push Up (3 in 1)		IST Alt. Side Step 2 Arm Chest Press

IST & THE BIG THREE

SQUAT DAY	BENCH DAY	DEADLIFT DAY
5x5 Front Squat	5x5 Bench Press	5x5 Deadlift
IST Forward Step Chest Press	IST Side Step Deadlift	IST Rear Rotation Step Squat
IST Rear Rotation Step Rotating Overhead Press	IST Rear Rotation Step Row	IST Forward Step Shoulder Press
IST Rear Step Ankle Height Row	IST Forward Step Curl to Chest Press	IST Rotation Step Chest Press

IST & PCC

DAY 1 CHEST/BICEPS	DAY 2 LEGS	DAY 3 BACK/TRICEPS	DAY 4 SHOULDER
IST - Alternating Forward Step Chest Press	IST - Alternating Side Step Squat Front Load	IST - IST Pull Up Complex	IST - Alternating Forward Step Shoulder Press
PCC - Archer Push Up	IST - Alternating Rear Step Deadlift	IST - Alternating Rear Step Ankle Height Row	PCC - Wall Stand, Handstand,
IST - Alternating Rear Step Bicep Curl	PCC - Pistol Squat	IST - Side Step With Triceps Ext. Across Body	IST - IST Push Up Complex
PCC - Elbow Lever	IST - Rear Rotation Step Deadlift	PCC - Archer Pull Up	IST - Rear Rotation Step Rotating Overhead Press
IST - Alternating Rear Rotation Step Double Bicep Curl	IST - Alternating Front Step Front Squat	IST - Rear Rotation Step Shoulder Height Row	PCC - Thoracic Bridge, Half Back Bridge, Full Back Bridge
IST - Side Step Rotation Chest Press	PCC - Forward Walking Crab	PCC - Pike Push Up	IST - Side Step Side Raise

IST 2 DAY SPLIT Each exercise should be done for a set of 8-12

DAY 1 CABLE HEIGHT (LOW)	DAY 2 CABLE HEIGHT (HIGH)
IST Rear Rotation Step Row - Front Facing	IST rear Rotation Step Curl to chest press - Side Facing
IST Rear Rotation Step Curl to Chest Press - Side Facing	IST rear rotation step row - Front Facing
IST Squat Combo (Rear Step & Side Step)	IST Deadlift Combo (Side step & Rear step)
IST Push up (3 in 1)	IST Pull Up

IST & RKC

DAY 1 CHEST/BICEPS	DAY 2 LEGS	DAY 3 BACK/TRICEPS	DAY 4 SHOULDER
RKC - Single Arm Kettlebell Deadlift	RKC - Single Arm Kettlebell Clean and Press	RKC - Kettlebell Front Squat (8,5,3)	RKC - Turkish Get-Up 5x1 Each Side
IST - IST Push Up Complex	IST - Rear Rotation Step Rotational Overhead Press	IST - Side Step Chest Press Across Body	IST - Rear Rotation Step with Row Pull Through
RKC - Single Arm Kettlebell Swings	RKC - Kettlebell Snatch	RKC - Renegade Row	RKC - 1 Arm Loaded Overhead Carry
IST - Alternating Forward Step Chest Press	IST - Alternating Rear Step Row	IST - IST Dip Complex	IST - IST Pull Up Complex

MOVING BUILDER FOUR DAY
Each exercise should be done for a set of 8-12

DAY 1 - CHEST AND BICEPS	DAY 2 - LEGS AND ABS	DAY 3 - BACK AND TRICEPS	DAY 4 - SHOULDERS
IST Alt. Forward Step ChestPress	IST Alt Rear Step Deadlift	IST Rear Step Pull Down	IST Forward Step Shoulder Activator
IST Alt Side Step Row		IST Alt Side Step Tricep Pushdown	Quadruped Crawl Side to Side
IST Push Up (3 in 1)	IST Rear Rotation Front Squat		
IST Pull Up (3 in 1) Under Grip	Quadruped Kick Throughs	IST Side Step Bent Over Row (under-hand grip)	IST Forward Step Overhead Press
		IST Forward Step Overhead Tricep Extension	Hanging Knee to Chest Raise
IST Side Step Chest Press to Midline	IST Alternating Side Squat Slide		
IST Alt Forward Step Bicep Curl (use dumbbell)	IST Plank Alt. Forward Step	IST Dips - 3 in 1	IST Side Step Side Shoulder Raise
		IST Pull lps - 3 in 1	IST Side Arm Step Plank
IST Alt. Forward Step Chest Fly	IST Rear Rotation Step Deadlift		
Rotational Crawl		IST Rear Rotation Row	IST Rear Rotation Step Rotating Press
	IST Forward Step Toe Squat	IST Side Step Tricep Extension Across Body	IST Side Foot Step Plank
IST Alt Rear Rotation Step Rope Curl	Pistol - 1 Leg Squat		
Hanging Knee to Chest Raises		Front Lever Swings - (ice cream scoop)	IST Alt Rear Step Row
			IST Rear Rotation Hand Step Plank
Frog Stand / Crow Pose Practice			L Sit Hold on Dip Bars

ABOUT THE AUTHOR

Angelo Grinceri has been featured in People, Galore, MSN, Yahoo, EatThisNotThat, Cheatsheet and Gear Patrol.

As a child, Angelo excelled at sports like biking, motocross, football, weight lifting, track, and cross country. During his high school years, he became obsessed with bodybuilding. Bodybuilding gave Angelo the body of a super hero, but without super hero abilities. He became too stiff to enjoy his favorite sports, too bulky to wear his favorite clothes, and suffered from chronic shoulder and back pain. Angelo finally realized that all of this muscle didn't translate to full body strength—he was only strong and comfortable on machines and in a single foot position at one time.

Angelo embarked on a new quest, studying pain management, compound and dynamic movement training, advanced calisthenics, movement screening, and holistic nutrition. After years of experimentation, he developed Intrinsic Strength Training (IST) as an answer to isolation-based resistance training.

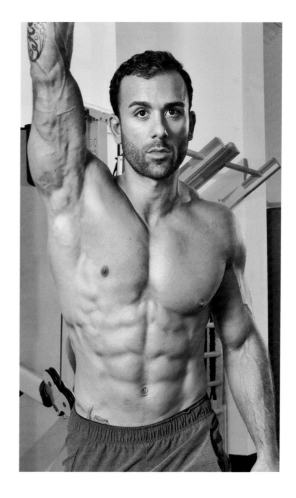

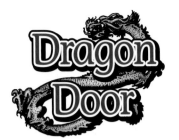

1·800·899·5111

24 HOURS A DAY • FAX YOUR ORDER (866) 280-7619

ORDERING INFORMATION

Telephone Orders For faster service you may place your orders by calling Toll Free 24 hours a day, 7 days a week, 365 days per year. When you call, please have your credit card ready.

Customer Service Questions? Please call us between 9:00am– 11:00pm EST Monday to Friday at 1-800-899-5111. Local and foreign customers call 513-346-4160 for orders and customer service

100% One-Year Risk-Free Guarantee. If you are not completely satisfied with any product—we'll be happy to give you a prompt exchange, credit, or refund, as you wish. Simply return your purchase to us, and please let us know why you were dissatisfied--it will help us to provide better products and services in the future. Shipping and handling fees are non-refundable.

Complete and mail with full payment to: Dragon Door Publications, 5 County Road B East, Suite 3, Little Canada, MN 55117

Please print clearly
Sold To: A

Name_____

Street_____

City_____

State_____ Zip_____

Day phone*_____

* Important for clarifying questions on orders

Please print clearly
Sold To: (Street address for delivery)   B

Name_____

Street_____

City_____

State_____ Zip_____

Email_____

Warning to foreign customers: The Customs in your country may or may not tax or otherwise charge you an additional fee for goods you receive. Dragon Door Publications is charging you only for U.S. handling and international shipping. Dragon Door Publications is in no way responsible for any additional fees levied by Customs, the carrier or any other entity.

ITEM #	QTY.	ITEM DESCRIPTION	ITEM PRICE	A OR B	TOTAL

HANDLING AND SHIPPING CHARGES • NO CODS

Total Amount of Order Add (Excludes kettlebells and kettlebell kits):

$00.00 to 29.99	Add $7.00	$100.00 to 129.99	Add $14.00
$30.00 to 49.99	Add $6.00	$130.00 to 169.99	Add $16.00
$50.00 to 69.99	Add $8.00	$170.00 to 199.99	Add $18.00
$70.00 to 99.99	Add $11.00	$200.00 to 299.99	Add $20.00
		$300.00 and up	Add $24.00

Canada and Mexico add $6.00 to US charges. All other countries, flat rate, double US Charges. See Kettlebell section for Kettlebell Shipping and handling charges.

Total of Goods	
Shipping Charges	
Rush Charges	
Kettlebell Shipping Charges	
OH residents add 6.5% sales	
tax	
MN residents add 6.5% sales	

METHOD OF PAYMENT ___CHECK ___M.O. ___MASTERCARD ___VISA ___DISCOVER ___AMEX

Account No. (Please indicate all the numbers on your credit card)   EXPIRATION DATE

▢▢▢▢ ▢▢▢▢▢ ▢▢▢▢▢ ▢▢▢▢ ▢▢ / ▢▢

Day Phone: _____

Signature: _____ Date: _____

NOTE: We ship best method available for your delivery address. Foreign orders are sent by air. Credit card or International M.O. only. **For RUSH processing** of your order, add an additional $10.00 per address. Available on money order & charge card orders only.

Errors and omissions excepted. Prices subject to change without notice.

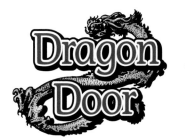

1·800·899·5111

24 HOURS A DAY • FAX YOUR ORDER (866) 280-7619

ORDERING INFORMATION

Telephone Orders For faster service you may place your orders by calling Toll Free 24 hours a day, 7 days a week, 365 days per year. When you call, please have your credit card ready.

Customer Service Questions? Please call us between 9:00am– 11:00pm EST Monday to Friday at 1-800-899-5111. Local and foreign customers call 513-346-4160 for orders and customer service

100% One-Year Risk-Free Guarantee. If you are not completely satisfied with any product—we'll be happy to give you a prompt exchange, credit, or refund, as you wish. Simply return your purchase to us, and please let us know why you were dissatisfied--it will help us to provide better products and services in the future. Shipping and handling fees are non-refundable.

Complete and mail with full payment to: Dragon Door Publications, 5 County Road B East, Suite 3, Little Canada, MN 55117

Please print clearly

Sold To: A

Name_____

Street_____

City_____

State_____ Zip_____

Day phone*_____
* Important for clarifying questions on orders

Please print clearly

Sold To: (Street address for delivery)   B

Name_____

Street_____

City_____

State_____ Zip_____

Email_____

Warning to foreign customers: The Customs in your country may or may not tax or otherwise charge you an additional fee for goods you receive. Dragon Door Publications is charging you only for U.S. handling and international shipping. Dragon Door Publications is in no way responsible for any additional fees levied by Customs, the carrier or any other entity.

ITEM #	QTY.	ITEM DESCRIPTION	ITEM PRICE	A OR B	TOTAL

HANDLING AND SHIPPING CHARGES • NO CODS

Total Amount of Order Add (Excludes kettlebells and kettlebell kits):

$00.00 to 29.99	Add $7.00	$100.00 to 129.99	Add $14.00
$30.00 to 49.99	Add $6.00	$130.00 to 169.99	Add $16.00
$50.00 to 69.99	Add $8.00	$170.00 to 199.99	Add $18.00
$70.00 to 99.99	Add $11.00	$200.00 to 299.99	Add $20.00
		$300.00 and up	Add $24.00

Canada and Mexico add $6.00 to US charges. All other countries, flat rate, double US Charges. See Kettlebell section for Kettlebell Shipping and handling charges.

Total of Goods	
Shipping Charges	
Rush Charges	
Kettlebell Shipping Charges	
OH residents add 6.5% sales	
tax	
MN residents add 6.5% sales	

METHOD OF PAYMENT ___CHECK ___M.O. ___MASTERCARD ___VISA ___DISCOVER ___AMEX

Account No. (Please indicate all the numbers on your credit card)   EXPIRATION DATE

▢▢▢▢ ▢▢▢▢ ▢▢▢▢ ▢▢▢▢   ▢▢/▢▢

Day Phone: _____

Signature: _____ Date: _____

NOTE: We ship best method available for your delivery address. Foreign orders are sent by air. Credit card or International M.O. only. **For RUSH processing** of your order, add an additional $10.00 per address. Available on money order & charge card orders only.

Errors and omissions excepted. Prices subject to change without notice.